Primer of
Sectional Anatomy with MRI and CT Correlation

Second Edition

Primer of
Sectional Anatomy with MRI and CT Correlation

Second Edition

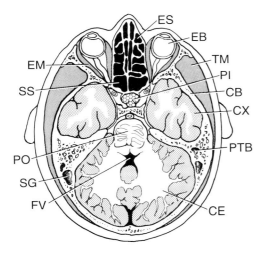

Charles P. Barrett, Ph.D.

Associate Professor of Anatomy
University of Maryland School of Medicine
Baltimore, Maryland

Larry D. Anderson, Ph.D.

Associate Professor of Anatomy
University of Maryland School of Medicine
Baltimore, Maryland

Lawrence E. Holder, M.D., F.A.C.R.

Professor of Radiology
Director, Division of Nuclear Medicine
University of Maryland Medical System
Baltimore, Maryland

Steven J. Poliakoff, M.D.

Assistant Professor of Anatomy
University of Maryland School of Medicine
Baltimore, Maryland

*With the special assistance of Kenneth R. Ballou B.S., C.N.M.T.
and William Parkent, B.S.*

Illustrations by Lydia Kibiuk

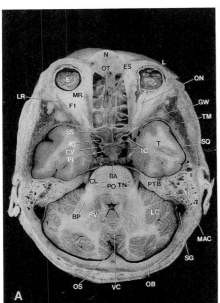

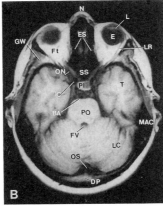

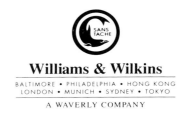

Williams & Wilkins

BALTIMORE • PHILADELPHIA • HONG KONG
LONDON • MUNICH • SYDNEY • TOKYO

A WAVERLY COMPANY

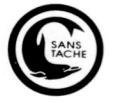

Editor: Pat A. Coryell
Managing Editor: Linda S. Napora
Copy Editor: Judith Minkove
Designer: Wilma Rosenberger
Illustration Planner: Wayne Hubbel
Production Coordinator: Anne G. Seitz

Copyright © 1994
Williams & Wilkins
428 East Preston Street
Baltimore, Maryland 21202, USA

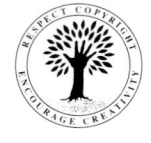

Accurate indications, adverse reactions, and dosage schedules for drugs are provided
in this book, but it is possible that they may change. The reader is urged to review the
package information data of the manufacturers of the medications mentioned.

Printed in the United States of America

First Edition 1990

Library of Congress Cataloging-in-Publication Data

Primer of sectional anatomy with MRI and CT correlation / Charles P. Barrett . . . [et
 al.] ; with the special assistance of Kenneth R. Ballou and William Parkent ; with
 illustrations by Lydia V. Kibiuk. — 2nd ed.
    p.   cm.
   Rev. ed of.: Primer of sectional anatomy with MRI and CT correlation / Charles
 P. Barrett, Steven J. Poliakoff, Lawrence E. Holder. c1990.
   Includes index.
   ISBN 0-683-00472-7
   1. Human anatomy—Atlases.   2. Magnetic resonance imaging—
Atlases.   3. Tomography—Atlases.   I. Barrett, Charles P.   II. Barrett,
Charles P.   Primer of sectional anatomy with MRI and CT correlation.
   [DNLM: 1. Anatomy, Regional—atlases.   2. Magnetic Resonance Imaging—
atlases.   3. Tomography, X-Ray Computed—atlases.   QS 17   P953 1994]
QM25.B323   1994
611'.0022'2—dc20
DNLM/DLC
for Library of Congress   93-34302
                                CIP

                   94 95 96 97 98
           1 2 3 4 5 6 7 8 9 10

To our children

Matthew, Julia, Brenda, Jennifer

Brent and Sheana

Annie, David, Elizabeth

Acknowledgments

This *Primer* would not have been possible without the help and encouragement of many people in several institutions. At the University of Maryland, Department of Anatomy, we especially thank William Parkent, B.S.; Jennifer Carandang; Fred Bland, B.S.; and Drs. Marshall Rennels, Rosemary Rees, and Judy Strum. Tammy Cohen was instrumental in the preparation of the manuscript. Ron Wade, B.S., Director of the State Anatomy Board and Joseph VanSant, senior embalmer, were also extremely helpful in locating anatomical specimens. Ken Ballou, B.S., C.N.M.T., of Sopha Medical Systems, was again tireless in his efforts to search out appropriate image correlations. Donna Haggerty, R.T., was also helpful in this regard. At the University of Maryland, Mardina Boykins, R.T.R., and Sheila O'Brien, R.T.R., were helpful with image acquisition. Our radiology colleagues at the University of Maryland included Drs. Kate Grumbaugh, Philip Hughes, Michael Rothman, and Charles White, and, at the Union Memorial Hospital, Baltimore, Dr. Andrew Yang, who answered many image correlation and clinical questions. Finally, we are extremely grateful to all of the people at Williams & Wilkins who worked patiently with us toward the completion of the *Primer*.

Contents

Chapter 3. **Abdomen**

Chapter 4.   *Pelvis*

Introduction

Diagnostic investigations and surgical procedures begin at the surface of the body. To perform either task well, clinicians must be able to visualize the arrangement of numerous structures that lie hidden from view beneath the surface. Acquisition of a working knowledge of this arrangement is most often gained by cadaver dissection. However, learning by dissection is useful only when the detail uncovered can be mentally resynthesized into a three-dimensional visualization of particular regions. This is readily accomplished by studying cadaver slices, since mental pictures developed in this way permit quick recall of many or all relevant anatomical relationships. There is yet another benefit. Studies of cadaver slices can be correlated with clinically equivalent magnetic resonance images (MRIs) and computerized tomographs (CT), thus affording an excellent opportunity for integration of basic anatomical science with clinical medicine.

New in the Second Edition

The primary format is the same for the Second Edition in that we continue to use labeled cadaver slices matched with comparable MR images or CT scans, which are also labeled. We have attempted to achieve close matches, but keep in mind that cadaver slices may deviate from the electronic images in terms of plane of section or because of varying physical characteristics between living patients and cadavers. Where this is significant, it is pointed out in the description of each plate. The second edition of the *Primer* has been rearranged and expanded and now contains 61 instead of 50 plates, arranged in five chapters instead of the original seven sections. We have greatly increased the number of identifying labels on all of the plates and have chosen to put the identifying labels on the plates, using initials. This has allowed us to use larger plate figures, which enables clearer visualization of structural detail.

Although we have increased the number of labels, we stress that improved understanding of sectional anatomy presented in the *Primer* will be better achieved by reference to more detailed anatomical atlases. For this reason, we continue to cite widely used atlases for each of the plates used in this *Primer*. A number of plates in the *Primer* are also cross-referenced to each other.

Other changes in this edition include revision of plate titles to more clearly define the important contents of individual body sections and to more specifically indicate the level of a particular section. Where appropriate, planes of transaxial sections include numbered vertebral levels. All of the original plates have been revised or replaced. Plates for the chapters on the head, thorax, and the female pelvis have been redone, using new cadaver slices and new MRI images, using state-of-the-art imaging software. The head is presented in orbitomeatal planes of section. A greatly expanded consideration of the extremities has been added, with all the major limb joints presented in two or more planes. We have also included a new section regarding the use of the *Primer*, which follows.

The index has been expanded to include the clinical terms. Furthermore, all terms are doubly indexed to ensure ease of finding the items mentioned in the text or identified on the plates.

How to Use This Primer

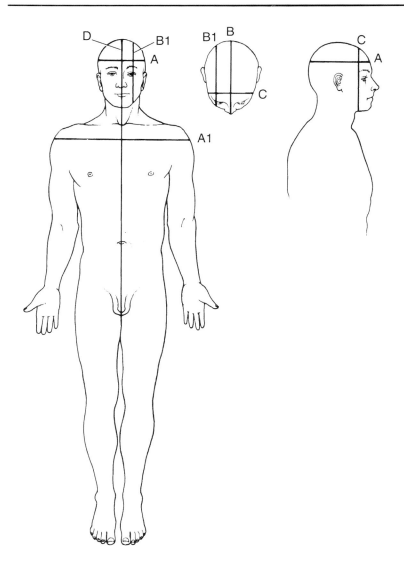

Figure 1. Transaxial, sagittal, and coronal planes of the body. *Transaxial planes* refer to planes that cut perpendicular to the axial line of the region being described. Planes **A** and **A1** are examples. Transaxial is preferred to the more general terms "cross" or "horizontal" when describing this plane of section. *Sagittal planes* refer to planes at or parallel to the median plane of the body (**D** in the figure). Planes **B** and **B1** are examples. *Coronal* or *frontal planes* refer to planes that are perpendicular to the median plane of the body. Plane **C** is an example. Note that the transaxial sectional modality is the most easily understood and is used clinically for MRI and CT procedures in all regions of the body. For these reasons, this modality is emphasized in this *Primer*.

Understanding the conventions used

The cadaver slices and electronic images in the *Primer* are in the transaxial, sagittal, and coronal planes, as explained in Figure 1 and as further detailed in the diagrams accompanying the plates. Levels of planes or the slight oblique variations from such planes are indicated in the diagram accompanying each plate.

Each plate, except the review plates, contains cadaver slices and electronic images. When feasible, structures visible in both the cadaver slices and electronic images are labeled. However, no attempt has been made to "force the anatomy" on the electronic images. When there is anatomical doubt or when the technique does not optimally demonstrate a structure, reference is made to the "region" of the particular structure.

Cadaver slices and electronic images used in the *Primer* are presented with the cadaver or patient in the anatomical position. As such, transaxial images and sections are oriented as if viewed from inferior, i.e., looking up from the cadaver's or patient's feet. Coronal slices and images are viewed from their anterior sides and sagittal ones from the lateral side.

The inclusion of numbered vertebral levels for structures in the thorax, abdomen, and pelvis warrants some caution. Levels of many organs vary from patient to patient due to respiratory fluctuations, size differences, degree of organ fullness, and body habitus and position. Similar variations occur in cadavers. On the average, however, most structures normally occupy relatively fixed vertebral levels ($\pm$ 1 to 2 segments) so that these levels are useful reference points. In individual bodies, most organs also tend to occupy constant positions relative to one another. Thus, images made at given spinal levels have good correspondence from patient to patient.

Awareness of organs present in section examined

As you begin the study of any region, your first question should be, "What are the major structures normally found in the region?" The global diagram presented in Figure 2 will help to establish the general outline of the principal contents as will observing the figures in references cited along with the plates in the *Primer*.

Pattern recognition

It is good practice to develop mental images of the major sectional patterns of various regions. Pattern recognition will quickly allow you to outline relative positions of organs and other structures in cadaver slices or electronic images and greatly assist you in assembling and assimilating details. Figure 2 accomplishes this by presenting an overview of the entire body in idealized sketches of 21 key transaxial sections meant to serve as a general guide for reference. As you study the photographic plates, recall of such major patterns will allow you to learn the components within slices more quickly.

Development of three-dimensional visualization of structures and their layout

The development of a three-dimensional visualization is achieved by mental assembly of sequential two-dimensional cadaver slices or electronic images. The sketches in Figure 2 are helpful in this regard, but more detail is found in the plates on the pages following. A greater advantage is gained in reviewing the plates of the head and limbs, since these regions are presented in three planes of section.

For organs or structures that pass consecutively through sequential slices, note changes in shape from slice to slice. Viewing and studying the changing patterns of various structures or organs in cadaver slices or electronic images allows you to mentally synthesize and visualize the complete design of a

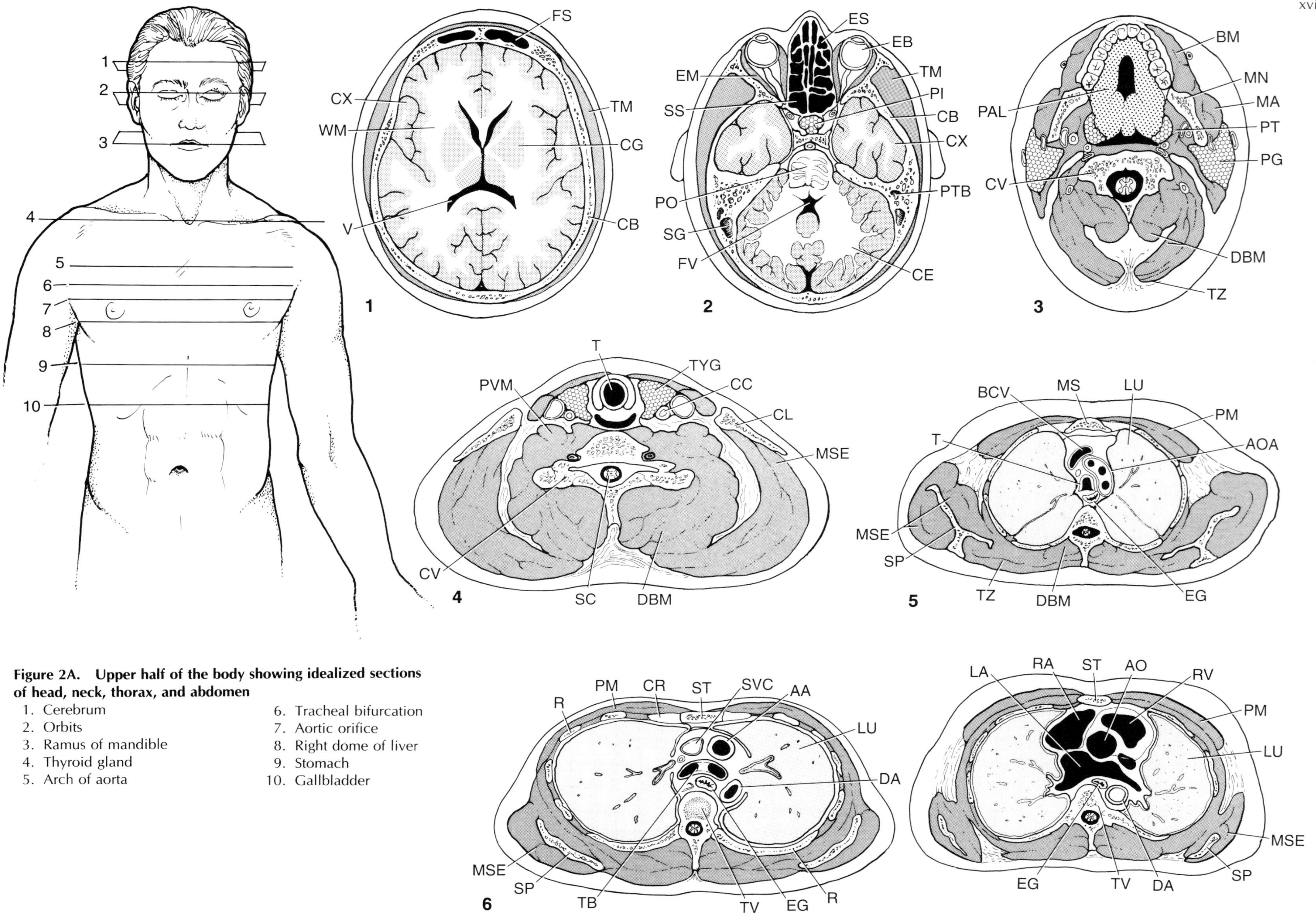

1
FS
CX
WM
TM
CG
V
CB

2
ES
EB
EM
SS
TM
PI
CB
CX
PO
SG
FV
PTB
CE

3
BM
MN
MA
PAL
PT
PG
CV
DBM
TZ

4
T
TYG
PVM
CC
CL
MSE
CV
SC
DBM

5
BCV
MS
LU
T
PM
AOA
MSE
SP
TZ
DBM
EG

6
R
PM
CR
ST
SVC
AA
LU
DA
MSE
SP
TB
TV
EG
R

LA
RA
ST
AO
RV
PM
LU
MSE
EG
TV
DA
SP

Figure 2A. Upper half of the body showing idealized sections of head, neck, thorax, and abdomen

1. Cerebrum
2. Orbits
3. Ramus of mandible
4. Thyroid gland
5. Arch of aorta
6. Tracheal bifurcation
7. Aortic orifice
8. Right dome of liver
9. Stomach
10. Gallbladder

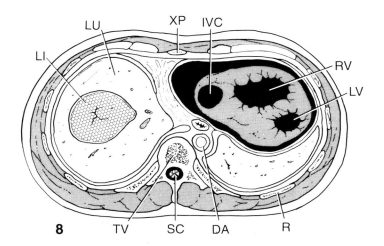

8

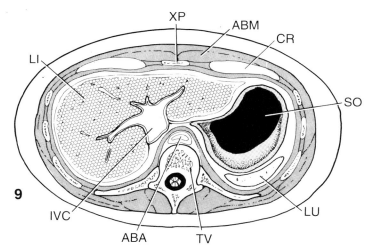

9

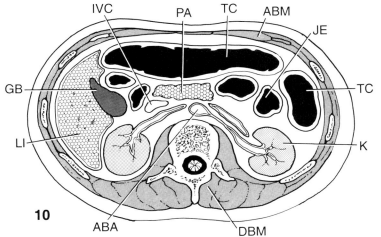

10

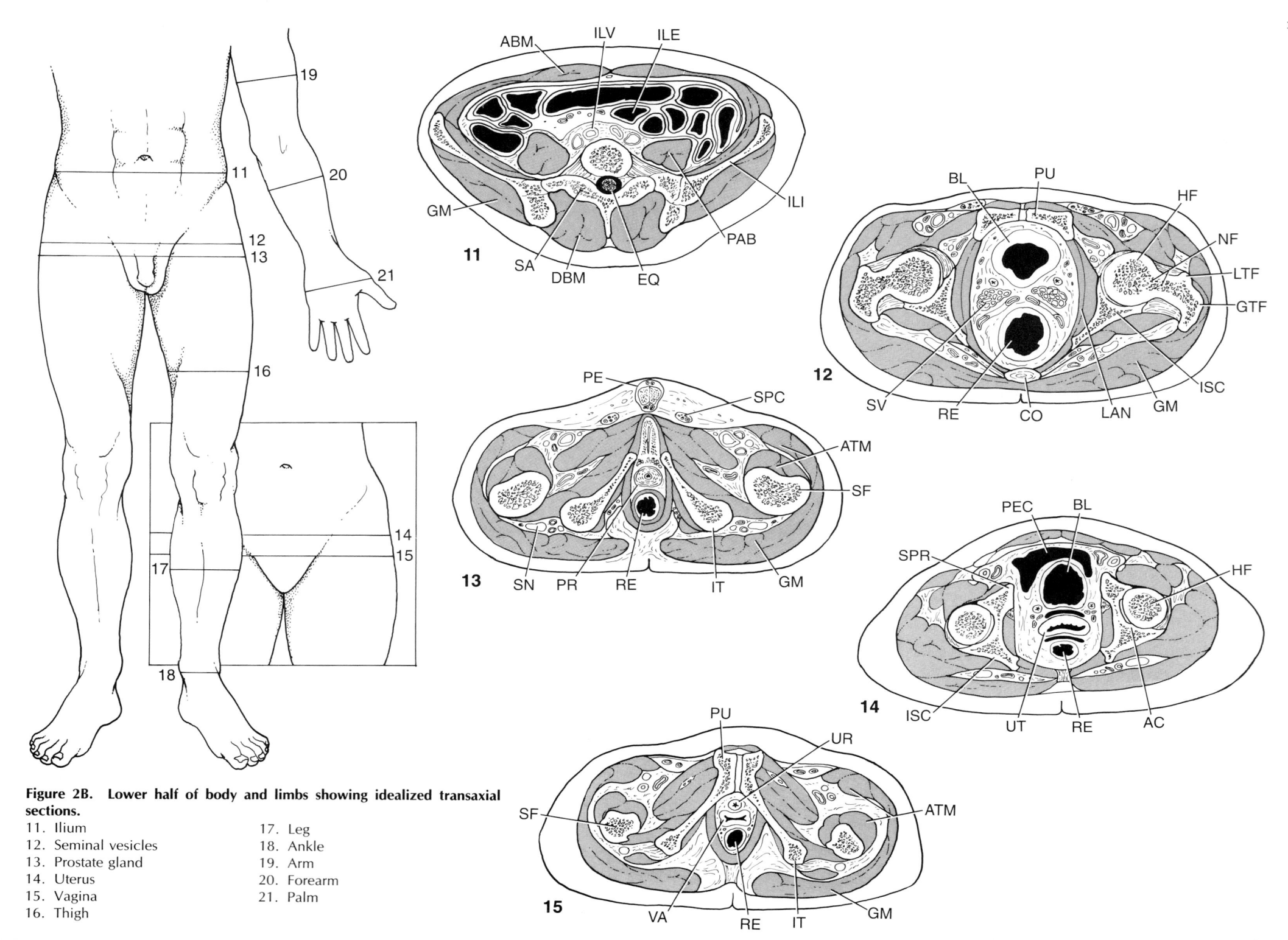

Figure 2B. Lower half of body and limbs showing idealized transaxial sections.

11. Ilium
12. Seminal vesicles
13. Prostate gland
14. Uterus
15. Vagina
16. Thigh
17. Leg
18. Ankle
19. Arm
20. Forearm
21. Palm

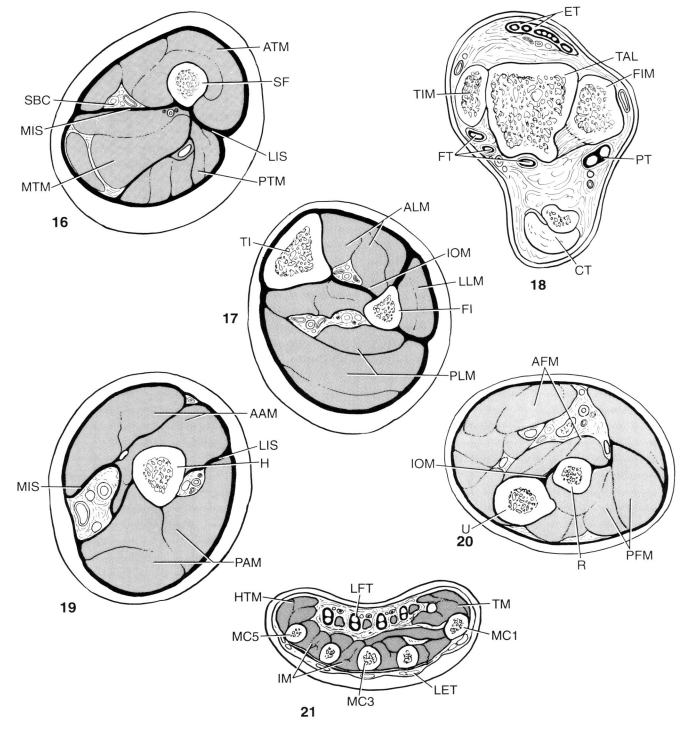

xix

given organ or structure, and through repetition of the process the complete structure of the region presented. In clinical practice, sequential images spaced 0.2 to 1 cm apart are commonly used to trace the longitudinal course of different structures and to evaluate the extent and location of tumors or other disease processes. For this reason and because this method is very useful for learning basic anatomy, we have inserted throughout the *Primer* a number of multiple photographs of sequential MR images or CT scans for review.

Developing a consistent way to study the plates

Develop a habit of observing the various parts of the section in a consistent order, such as that presented in the description of each plate. Note that these descriptions are primarily related to the wet specimens, which should therefore be studied first. The narrative descriptions are generally self-limited, and can be read over once or twice before you actually look at the plate.

Form a mental checklist as you study the morphological appearance of each structure, consciously relating it to its surrounding structures by reading the description with each plate to establish a more specific picture of the anatomical contents and their arrangement. After you feel satisfied that you are thoroughly familiar with the structural layout, proceed to one of the reference atlases and fill in as many details as you or your instructor desire.

Atlases that we have referenced include *Grant's Atlas of Anatomy, 9th edition*, Anne Agur, ed. (Baltimore: Williams & Wilkins, 1991); *Color Atlas of Anatomy, 2nd edition*, Johannes W. Rohen and Chirhior Yokochi (New York, Igaku-Shoin), and *Atlas of Anatomy*, Frank Netter, ed. (CIBA). The letter "G" referring to *Grant's Atlas* is followed by the chapter and figure number. For example, **G** 1-7 indicates Chapter 1, Figure 7. Similarly, the letters "RY" stand for Rohen-Yokochi, and "N" for Netter, followed by the page number.

Make use of the different planes of section in your studies. Transaxial sections reveal anterior, posterior, medial, lateral relations; coronal sections reveal medial, lateral, superior, and inferior relations; sagittal sections reveal anterior, posterior, superior, and inferior relations. The usefulness of observing different planes cannot be overemphasized.

If cadaver slices are available in your laboratory or dissection suite, compare the photographs in the *Primer* to them. By observing the pattern for given sections of a region, relationships of organs to one another will be more readily appreciated and visualized. Preview of cadaver slices along with the *Primer* will also greatly aid in orientation prior to dissection of given regions.

Enhanced understanding of anatomical structure through electronic imaging

Often, structural detail is made clearer by the characteristics of images obtained electronically. Make use of the varying signal characteristics of tissues in MR images or CT scans to assist you in differentiating between organs or structural components.

Magnetic resonance (MR) imaging is the correlative imaging modality predominantly used in this book. Conceptually quite different from x-ray imaging techniques, images can be produced in any plane, but are most often displayed in standard sagittal, coronal, and transaxial projections. However, in the clinical setting it is sometimes advantageous to display relationships in an oblique plane. When an anatomic structure such as the rotator cuff musculature in the shoulder is oblique to these planes, the images can be reconstructed and displayed obliquely to visualize more of a given structure in a single image.

MR imaging records data based upon the magnetic properties of hydrogen nuclei, which can be thought of as tiny magnets spinning in random directions. These nuclei (magnets) interact with neighboring atoms and with externally applied magnetic fields. When an outside source of strong magnetic energy

T1-weighted	T2-weighted
Bright, high-signal intensity	**Bright, high-signal intensity**
1 Fat	CSF, water 1
2 Marrow	2
3	3
4	Intervertebral disk 4
5 Brain, white matter	Brain, gray matter 5
6	6
7 Liver, pancreas	Spleen 7
8 Brain, gray matter	8
9 Kidney	9
10 Spleen	10
11	11
12	Brain, white matter 12
13	Liver 13
14 Cerebrospinal fluid	Fat 14
15 Water, lung	Iron in basal ganglia 15
16 Cortical bone, flowing blood, air	Bone, flowing blood, air 16
Dark, low-signal intensity	**Dark, low-signal intensity**

Figure 3. Comparison of signal intensities in data generated by T1 vs. T2 weighting.

is applied to these small magnetic fields, they are redirected to lie parallel to the direction of the external magnet. Radio waves from a secondary coil are then directed at the nuclei from another angle. The nuclei absorb this energy and flip 180° from their previous positions. Cessation of the secondary pulse results in a gradual return of the nuclei to their original, parallel state imposed by the magnet. The energy released during this process of nuclear redirection is measured electronically and analyzed by sophisticated computer algorithms to create a two-dimensional image depicting a thin tissue slice. Depending on their chemical environment, atoms require different amounts of energy to flip and require different times to return to their original orientation. For example, hydrogen in water emits a different spectrum than hydrogen in protein or fat. Since water and fat content varies from tissue to tissue or between a collection of tumor cells surrounding normal cells, differences in released energy can also be used to diagnose the presence of abnormalities within organs. T1 and T2 relaxation times are two measures of these energy-absorbing and -releasing characteristics. By altering parameters associated with data generation, images can be produced that emphasize either of these characteristics. In this *Primer*, the images have been created using T1 or T2 characteristics of the tissues, called T1 or T2 weighting. The relative gray scale positions of various tissues, when data are obtained with T1 or T2 weighting, are illustrated in Figure 3. MR parameters can also be altered to emphasize particular tissues such as cartilage or to evaluate blood flow without the use of contrast agents. These specialized techniques are beyond the scope of this *Primer*.

The other imaging modality used in this *Primer*, computed or computerized tomography (CT scanning), is based on x-ray technology. In standard radiography, the patient is positioned between x-rays from an x-ray source and a film sensitive to radiation. X-ray photons entering the patient are absorbed in proportion to relative densities of various tissue components. Emerging x-rays, variably absorbed and so with variable energies, expose the film to cause varying densities from clear to black. In this imaging modality, clear areas represent radiopaqueness (metal, bone-high absorbence) and darker ones represent radiolucency (water, fat, air-low absorbence). In computed tomography, x-ray photons interact with a scintillation crystal that is more sensitive than x-ray film. Sophisticated computers and programs applying algorithms similar to those used for MR imaging generate representative transaxial images. Display of CT images generally reflects the gradation between four basic densities: *air* (black), *fat* (dark/gray), *water/ blood* (light/gray), and *bone/metal* (white). Currently, CT scanning is the method of choice for overview abdominal studies, since patients are usually able to hold their breath for the 2 seconds of data acquisition required for each slice, thus eliminating the image degradation associated with respiratory motion. Refinements in data acquisition parameters and coils for MR imaging are reducing the time to acquire abdominal images so that even now, special questions about abdominal structures are studied using MRI. Most often, the choice of which imaging modality to use, is dictated by the nature of the tissue under examination. For example, bone marrow can be better characterized on MR images than on CT scans. However, bone detail is better seen on CT scans.

Miscellaneous items

Abbreviations used to identify structures were chosen to hint at the item being identified as much as possible. When a structure is described in the narrative text, its abbreviation follows and appears in italics.

Preparation of Anatomical Specimens

The anatomical specimens used in this *Primer* were prepared by freezing embalmed cadavers and sectioning them with a bandsaw. Following sectioning, specimens were further prepared by washing them under a stream of warm water and, in most cases, dissecting blood and other material from vessels and hollow organs before photography.

PLATE 1. Middle nasal concha, pituitary gland, and fourth ventricle: T1 MR image

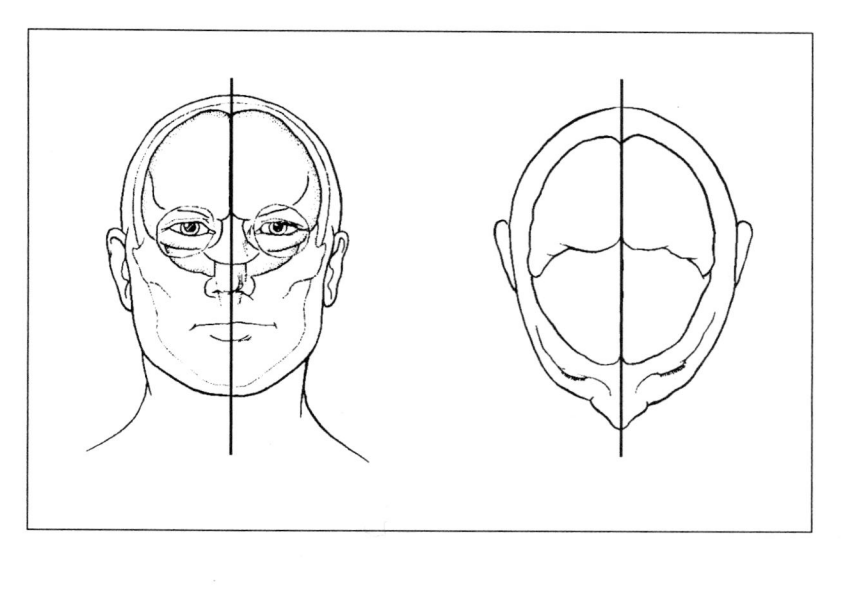

Note

- The **frontal** (F), **parietal** (P), and **occipital** (O) lobes of the cerebrum are roofed over by the calvaria represented here by the **frontal** (FB), **parietal** (PB), and **occipital bones** (OB).
- The **frontal sinus** (FS) lies above the **nasal cavity** (NC) in the **frontal bone** (FB) and, being air-filled, presents with a low (dark) signal in **B**.
- The **falx cerebri** (FC) seen only in **A** extends inferiorly from the **superior sagittal sinus** (SSS) between the left and right cerebral hemispheres.
- The **genu** (G), **body** (B), and **splenium** (S) of the corpus callosum arch above the **septum pellucidum** (SP), an artifactual hole that opens into the body of the right lateral ventricle (LV2).
- Centrally located diencephalic structures include the **third ventricle** (TV) here labeled on its lateral wall, **optic nerve** (ON), **infundibular stalk** (ID), **pituitary gland (hypophysis)** (PI), and **pineal gland (epithalamus)** (EP). The hypophyseal fossa in which the **pituitary gland** (PI) lies indents the posterior part of the roof of the **sphenoid sinus** (SS).
- Caudal to the diencephalic structures are the **mesencephalon (midbrain)** (MB), **pons** (PO), **medulla oblongata** (ME), and **cervical spinal cord** (C). The **dura mater** (DM) lines the vertebral canal, forming a sac that contains the cord and cerebrospinal fluid (CSF).
- The **basilar artery** (BA), formed by the vertebral arteries, lies posterior to the **clivus** (CL) and anterior to the **pons** (PO). In **B** the bright signal of fat in the marrow of the **clivus** (CL) is labeled.
- The floor of the **fourth ventricle** (FV) lies on the dorsum of the **pons** (PO) and the **medulla** (ME). This ventricle is related posteriorly to the **cerebellum** (CE).
- The **cerebellomedullary cistern (cisterna magna)** (CM) occupies the region of the **foramen magnum** (*white dots*) just inferior to the cerebellum.
- Immediately inferior to the foramen magnum the **dens (odontoid process)** (D) articulates with the posterior aspect of the **anterior arch of the atlas** (AA).
- Structures related to the oral cavity include the **mentis of the mandible** (MN4), **genioglossus** (GG), and the **mylohyoid** (MH) muscles.

Clinical Notes

- In T1 MR images, compact or cortical bone has a dark (low) signal, while marrow filled cancellous bone has a brighter (intermediate) signal. In this MR image, note the marrow and compact bone signals from the calvaria, hard palate, clivus, dens, and mandible. Reduction of signal intensity from marrow is often a sign of metastatic disease.
- Midline sagittal MR imaging is excellent for visualization of pituitary gland tumors, which may extend superiorly and impinge on the optic chiasma or inferiorly to invade the sphenoid sinus.
- The cervicomedullary junction is surrounded by the premedullary cistern and the cisterna magna and may be compressed from bone disease, tumors, or herniation of the cerebellar tonsil due to elevated intracranial pressure.
- The pineal gland, usually insignificant clinically, often presents as a calcified midline structure on plain radiographs or CT scans.
- Dura mater when sliced on edge appears as a thin intermediate signal, as seen in **B**.

References G *7-19, 7-106, 7-108, 7-109, 8-84, 8-85;* **N** *30, 43, 57;* **RY** *86, 90, 148*

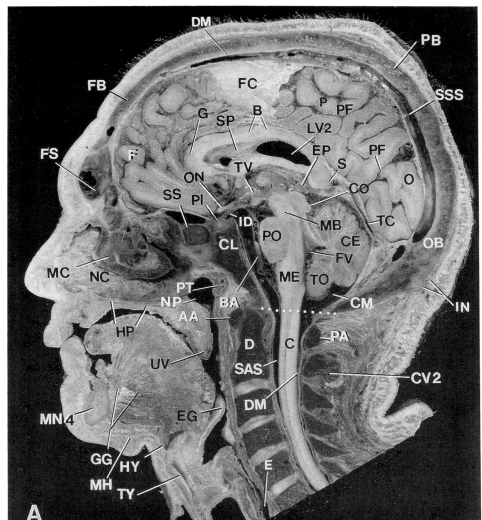

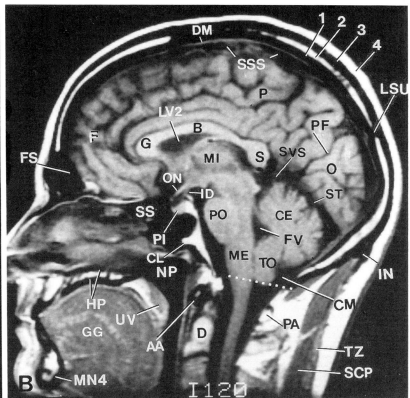

2

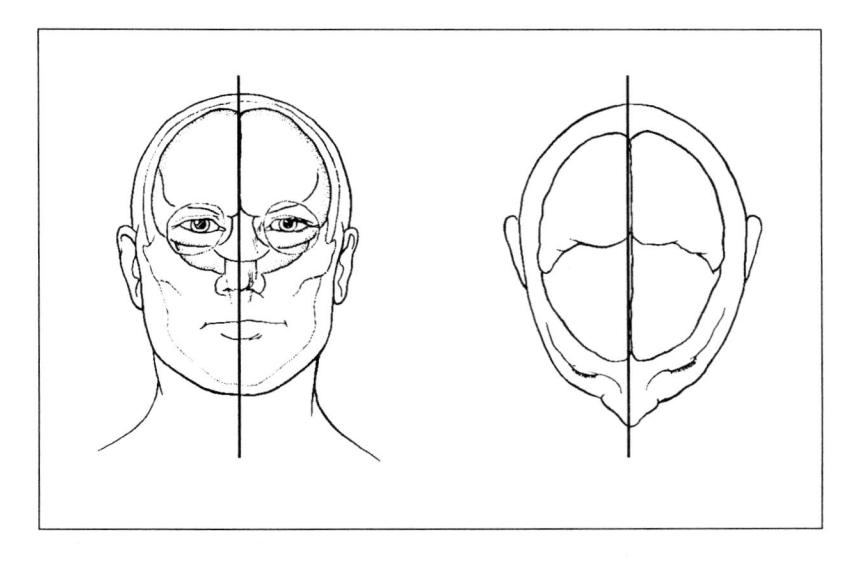

Note

- The **mentis of the mandible** (*MN4*) lies anteriorly and serves as an attachment for three muscles seen here: **genioglossus** (*GG*) passing into the **tongue** (*TG*), and **geniohyoid** (*GH*) and **mylohyoid** (*MH*) passing into the **hyoid bone** (*HY*).
- Structures forming an arc above the dorsum of the tongue include the **hard palate** (*HP*), **uvula** (*UV*), and, posteriorly at the root of the tongue, the **epiglottis** (*EG*).
- Inferior to the **epiglottis** (*EG*), the posterior wall of the **larynx** (*LX*) is anterior to the **pharynx** (*PH*), whose wall consists of the **superior** (*1*), **middle** (*2*), and **inferior** (*3*) constrictor muscles.
- The **anterior arch of the atlas** (*AA*) articulates with the **dens** (*D*) posterior to which is the **cervical spinal cord** (*C*), surrounded by **dura mater** (*DM*) and the **subarachnoid space** (*SAS*). Other central nervous system structures seen here include the **pons** (*PO*) and more caudally, the **medulla oblongata** (*ME*).
- The **fourth ventricle** (*FV*) has the **pons** (*PO*) and the **medulla** (*ME*) as its floor and the **cerebellum** (*CE*) as its roof.
- The **cerebellomedullary cistern (cisterna magna)** (*CM*) adjoins the **foramen magnum** (*white dots*).

Clinical notes

- T1 MR images reveal degeneration or herniation of intervertebral disks, allowing for cord or nerve root impingement to be identified and diagnosed.
- In T1 MR images, vertebral marrow and cortical bone have different signal intensities, i.e., bright vs. dark. The marrow signal darkens with the presence of infection or tumor as the normal fat content is replaced.

References **G** *8-84, 8-85;* **N** *30, 57;* **RY** *86, 90, 151*

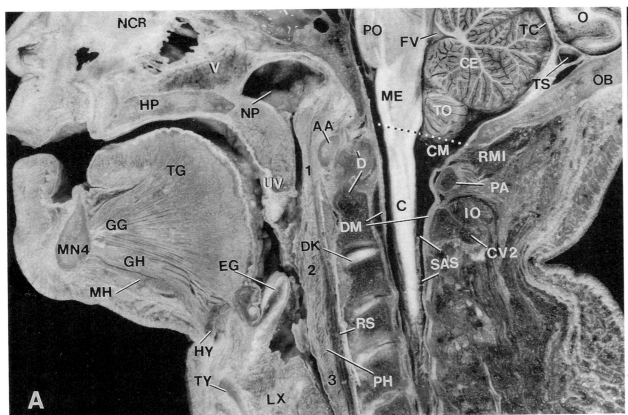

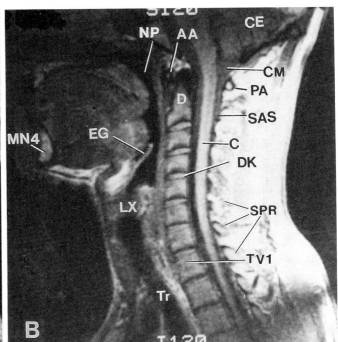

4

PLATE 3. Inferior nasal concha, ethmoid sinuses, and splenium of the corpus callosum: T1 MR image

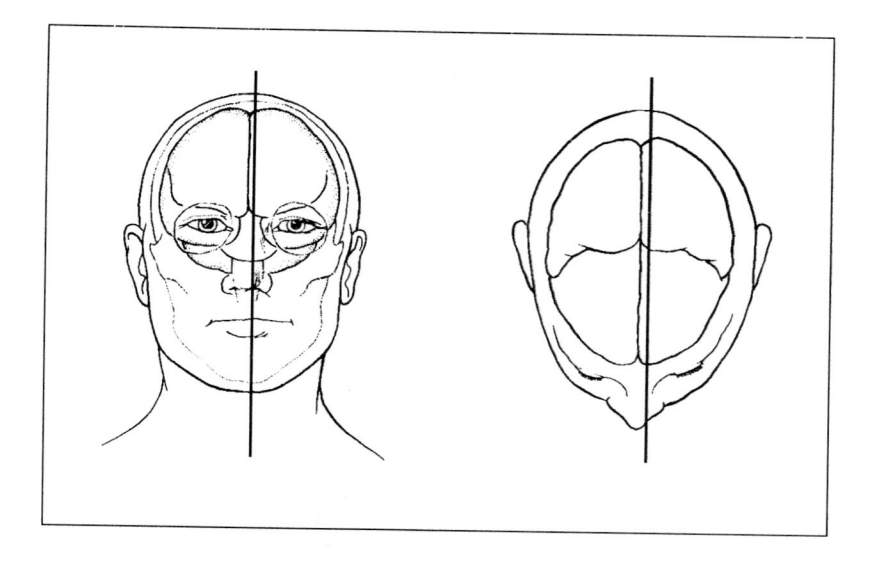

Note

- The **frontal** (*F*), **parietal** (*P*), and **occipital** (*O*) lobes of the cerebrum are covered by calvarial bones with corresponding names, as in Plate 1. The **tentorium cerebelli** (*TC*) separates the **occipital lobe** (*O*) from the **cerebellum** (*CE*). The **middle cerebral peduncle (brachium pontis)** (*MPO*) extends from the **pons** (*PO*) into the cerebellum.
- Deep CNS structures appear in the middle of the plate and include parts of the central gray matter, e.g., **caudate nucleus** (*CN*) and **red nucleus** (*RN*) as well as the **internal capsule** (*ICP*), the **body of the lateral ventricle** (*LV2*), and **genu** (*G*), **body** (*B*), and **splenium** (*S*) of the corpus callosum.
- The **frontal sinus** (*FS*) of the frontal bone lies anterior to the ethmoid bone containing the **ethmoid sinuses** (*ES*) just behind which is the **internal carotid artery** (*IC*) in the carotid canal. Inferior to the **ethmoid sinuses** (*ES*) is the nasal cavity with its **inferior nasal concha** (*ICo*).
- Structures related to the oral cavity and floor of the mouth include the tongue, **mentis of the mandible** (*MN4*), **genioglossus** (*GG*), and **mylohyoid** (*MH*).

Clinical Notes

- With aging, cerebral parenchyma often atrophies, and the sulci increase in size. The increase is detected by MR imaging.
- Some of the basal ganglia such as the caudate nucleus lie inferior to the lateral ventricle on sagittal sections. Hemorrhage or lacunar infarction is well delimited in these structures in MR images.

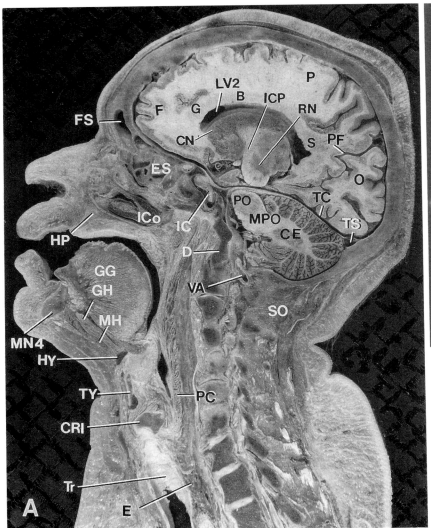

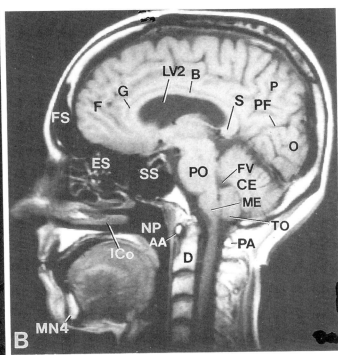

PLATE 4. Pterygoid process, hippocampus, and posterior (occipital) horn of the lateral ventricle: T1 MR image

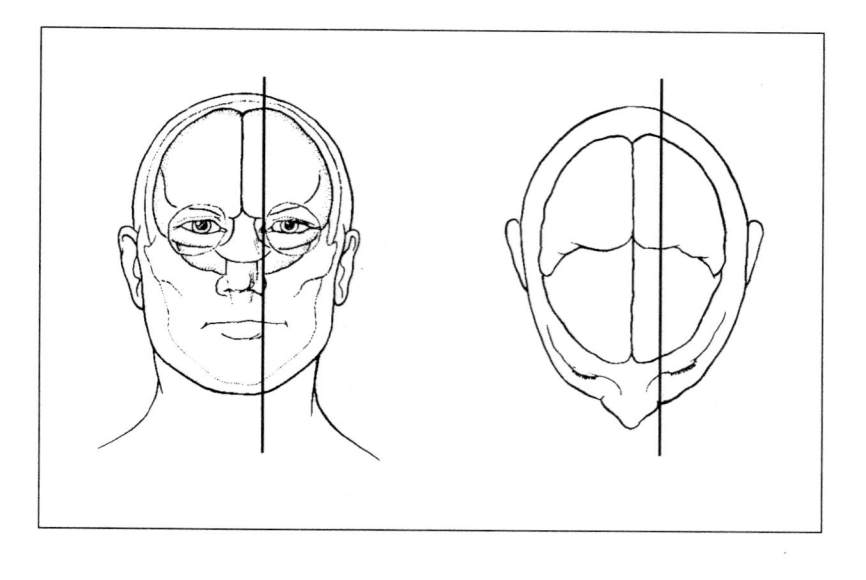

Note

- The MR image is slightly lateral to the wet specimen.
- The **frontal** (*F*), **parietal** (*P*), and **occipital** (*O*) lobes of the cerebrum are covered by bones with corresponding names, as in Plate 1. The **tentorium cerebelli** (*TC*) separates the **occipital lobe** (*O*) from the **cerebellum** (*CE*).
- Deep CNS structures appear in the middle of the plate and include a part of the basal ganglia: **putamen** (*PU*), the **corona radiata** (*CRA*), **internal capsule** (*ICP*), **body of the lateral ventricle** (*LV2*), **optic tract** (*OT*).
- At the posterior aspect of the orbit is the **optic nerve** (*ON*). Two extraocular muscles, **superior** and **inferior rectus** (*SR, IR*), stand out because their signal intensities are lower (darker) than the surrounding higher (bright) signal of the **intraorbital fat** (*Ft*) in **B**.
- The orbit is superior to the **maxillary sinus** (*MS*), which itself is superior to the **hard palate** (*HP*).
- Structures related to the oral cavity and floor of the mouth include the tongue, **mentis of the mandible** (*MN4*), **hyoid bone** (*HY*), the **sternohyoid** (*SH*) and the **mylohyoid** (*MH*).
- The dark region, designated *TE* in **B** arises from the presence of the **teeth,** which give a low-intensity signal.

Clinical Notes

- Intraorbital lesions can be located with respect to the low-intensity signal from the eyeball (black) and the high-intensity signal from the intraorbital fat (white).
- Air in sinuses and flowing blood, as in the vertebral artery, have low-signal (dark) intensities on T1 MR images. Magnetic resonance angiography (MRA) detects flowing blood without the need to inject intravenous contrast, as is required for radiographic angiograms.

References B *243;* **G** *7-117, 7-118, 7-50, 7-54*

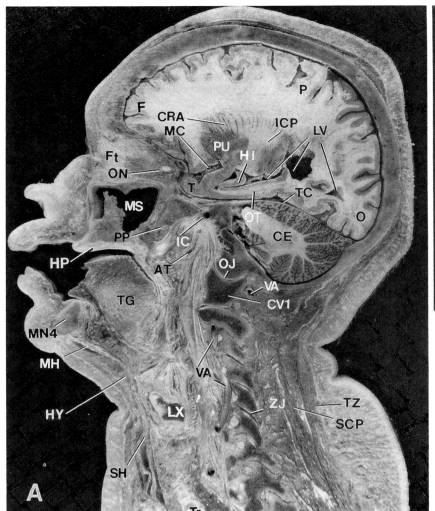

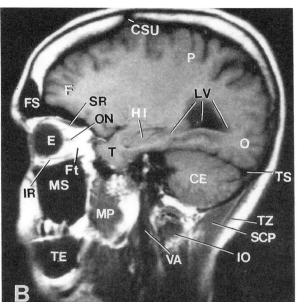

PLATE 5. Orbit, temporal lobe, and lateral lobe of cerebellum: T1 MR image

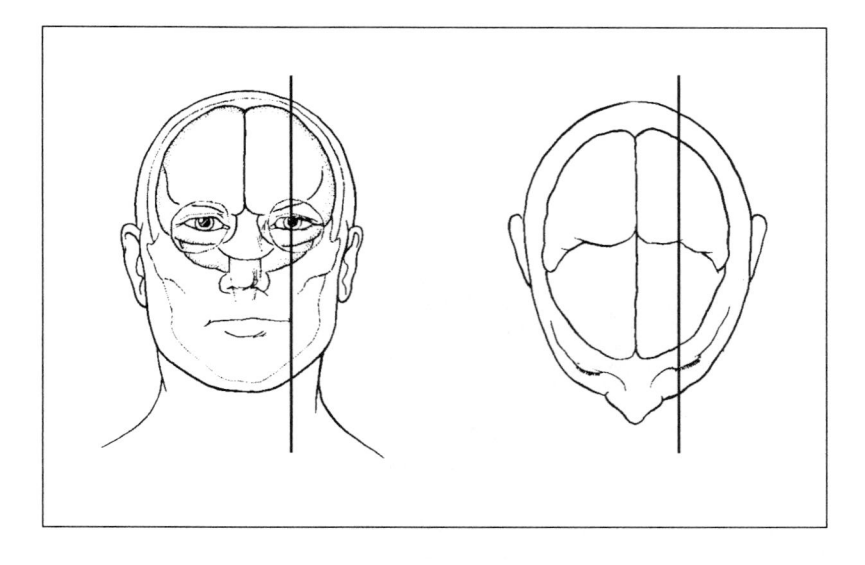

Note

- The MR image is more lateral than the wet specimen.
- The **frontal** (*F*), **parietal** (*P*), and **occipital** (*O*) lobes of the cerebrum are covered by bones with corresponding names, as in plate 1. The **tentorium cerebelli** (*TC*) separates the occipital lobe from the **cerebellum** (*CE*). The **lateral or sylvian fissure** (*LF*) separates the frontal and temporal lobes.
- The **lateral pterygoid** (*LP*) can be seen in the infratemporal region.
- The **parotid gland** (*PG*) appears posterior to the **ramus of the mandible** (*MN2*) and in confluent with the **submandibular gland** (*SMG*) inferior to the mandible. In **B** the **internal jugular vein** (*IJ*) lies in immediate relationship to the **parotid gland** (*PG*).
- Structures related to the oral cavity and floor of the mouth include the tongue and the **mandibular ramus** (*MN2*).

Clinical Notes

- The location of a lesion as either suprasylvian (frontal or parietal lobes) or infrasylvian (temporal lobe) determines the appropriate neurosurgical approach. As will be seen, the lateral or sylvian fissure is well demarcated by sagittal MR imaging.
- The temporal lobe abuts bone of the middle cranial fossa and is there subject to contusions in deceleration injuries.

*References **G** 7-50, 7-54, 7-61, 7-76; **N** 66; **R** 81, 82*

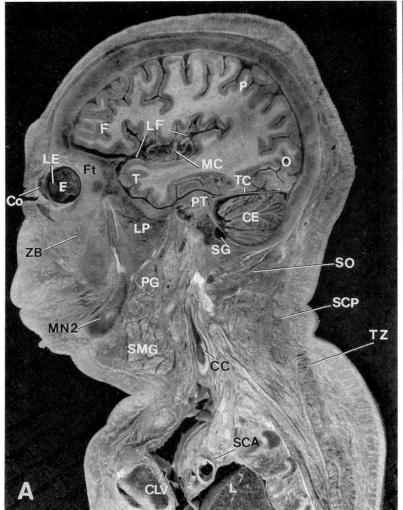

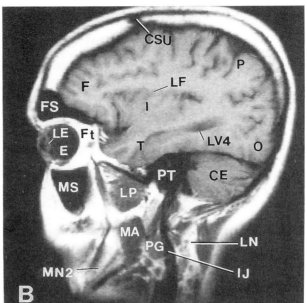

Chapter I. Head and Neck
Part I. Sagittal Sections

PLATE 6. Buccinator muscle, greater wing of sphenoid bone, and temporomandibular joint: T1 MR image

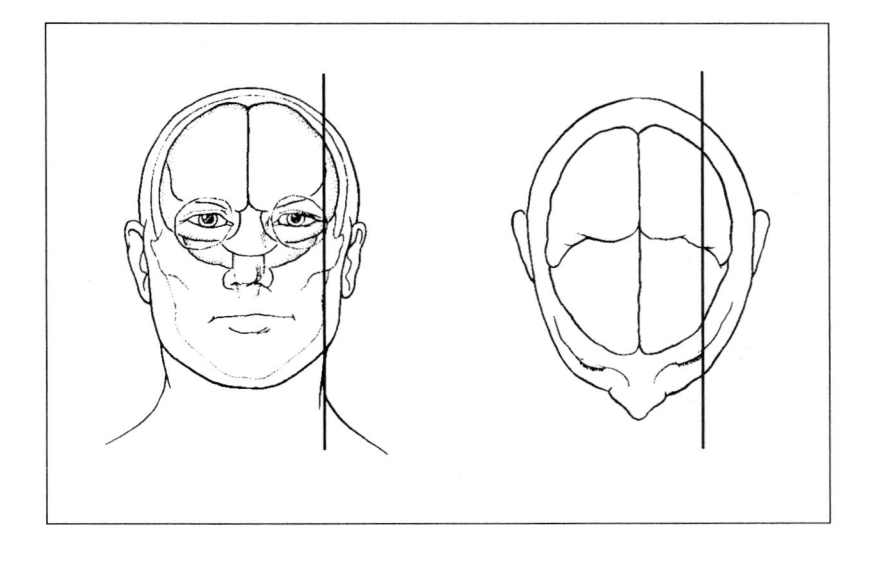

Note

- The MR image is slightly medial to the wet specimen.
- The **frontal** (*F*), **parietal** (*P*), and **occipital** (*O*) lobes of the cerebrum are covered by calvarial bones with corresponding names, as in plate 1. The **cerebellum** (*CE*) is out of the plane of section in **A** but appears in **B**. The **lateral (sylvian) fissure** (*LF*) separates the **frontal** (*F*) and **temporal** (*T*) cerebral lobes.
- The **parotid gland** (*PG*) is posterior to the neck **and head of the mandible** (*MN1*). Anterior to the neck, the inserting fibers of the **lateral pterygoid** (*LP*) are seen. The **disk** (*DK*) of the temporomandibular joint is also seen in its relationship to the neck and head of the mandible.
- Structures related to the oral cavity and floor of the mouth include the **buccinator** (*BU*), which forms the lateral wall of the mouth.
- The important relationships around the root of the neck and the thoracic cavity are evident in this section. The apex of the **lung** (*L*), **pleural cavity** (*PLC*), **subclavian artery** and **vein** (*SCA, SCV*), **clavicle** (*CLV*), and **first rib** (*R1*) are seen.

Clinical Notes

- The normal or abnormal parotid gland is well shown by T1 MR imaging.
- Trauma or disease of the parotid gland may compress or destroy branches of the facial nerve within it, resulting in paralysis of facial muscles.

*References **G** 7-61, 7-67, 7-76, 7-77; **N** 49, 55; **RY** 76-77*

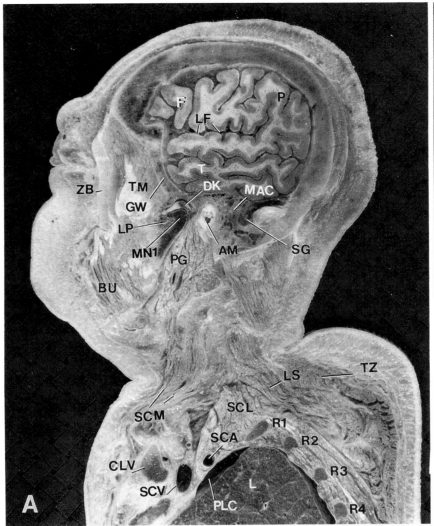

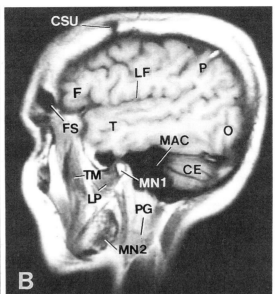

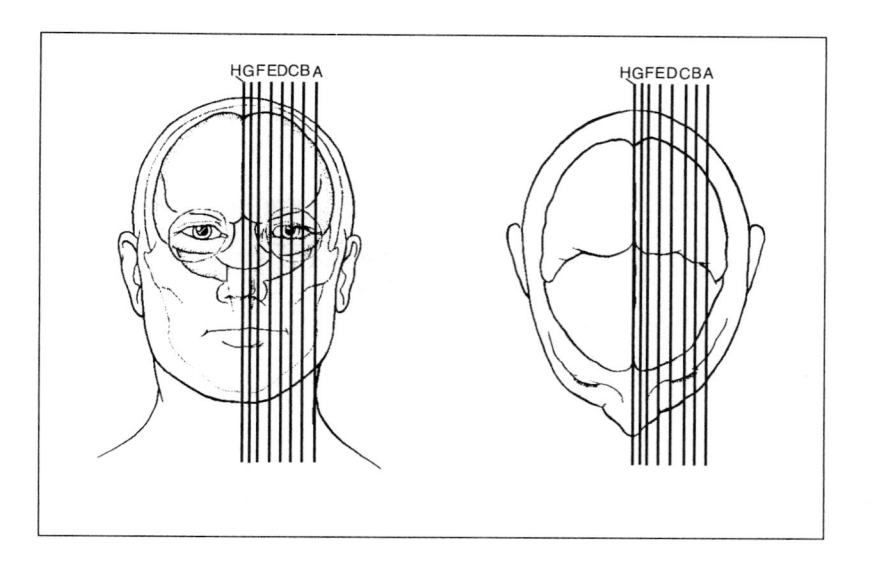

Note

A review of the plate below emphasizes the usefulness of sequential images in following the course of anatomic structures. Referring to this plate and to previous plates, it is possible to trace the changing form and extent of structures in a lateral **A** to medial **H** progression. The MR images here fall into various regions of the deep face and the cranium, and a few examples can be cited.

In **A**, two of the muscles of mastication, **lateral pterygoid** (*LP*) and the **temporalis** (*TM*) appear. Slightly more medially, in **B**, the **masseter** (*MA*) makes its appearance, and in **C,** the **medial pterygoid** (*MP*) is seen. In this same course, the **maxillary sinus** (*MS*) is seen in **B-F** anterior to the infratemporal region. The **frontal sinus** (*FS*) is seen concurrently and appears in **A-H**. As the **maxillary sinus** (*MS*) disappears towards the midline, the **sphenoid sinus** (*SS*) in **D-H**, and posterior to it, the **ethmoid sinus** (*ES*) in **F-G** appears. The midline aspect of the **sphenoid sinus** (*SS*), indented posterosuperiorly by the hypophyseal fossa containing the **pituitary gland (hypophysis)** (*PI*) is best seen in **H**. As another example, the extent of the **lateral ventricle** is traceable from its **anterior (frontal) horn** (*LV1*) in **E**, closest to the **head of the caudate nucleus** (*CN*), through its **body** (*LV2*) in **C-H**, through its **posterior (occipital) horn** (*LV3*) in **D-E** and the more lateral position of its **inferior (temporal) horn** (*LV4*) in **B**.

Clinical Notes

In clinical evaluation of the craniofacial region, size, extent, relationship and relative tissue characteristics of various structures are all important diagnostic considerations. In practice, MR or CT images are reviewed in sequences such as the sagittal one presented here. By referring to a series of images such as this, organs or structures are visualized through their extent. An orthogonal sequence, combining sagittal images with coronal or transaxial images, further aids visualization of the structure or lesion (abnormality) in its third dimension.

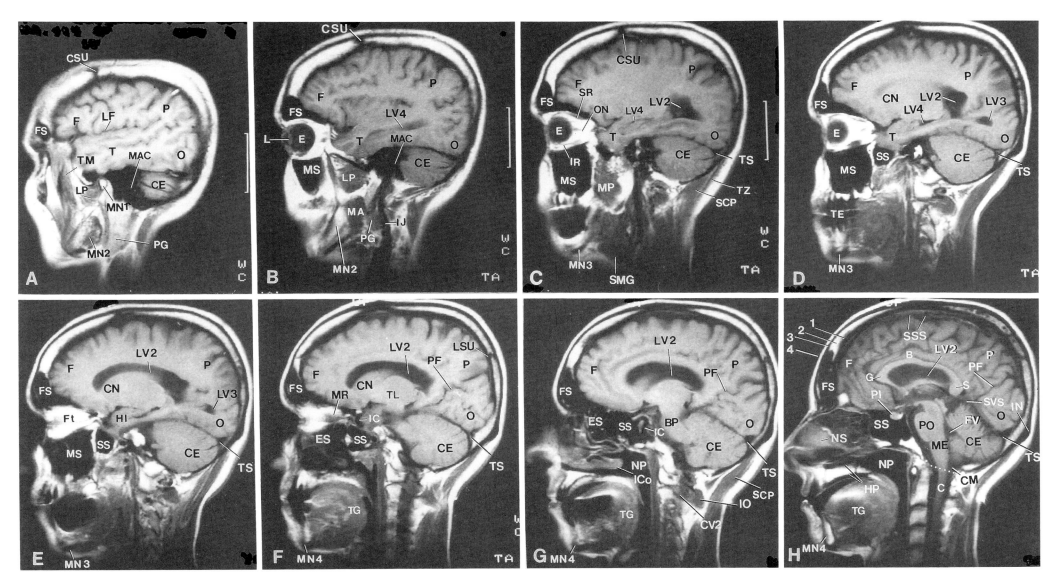

KEY

1 inner table of calvaria
2 diplöe
3 outer table of calvaria
4 subcutaneous fat of scalp
B body of corpus callosum
BP brachium pontis
C spinal cord
CE cerebellum
CM cisterna magna
CN head of caudate nucleus
CSU coronal suture
CV2 spine, cervical vertebra 2

E eyeball
ES ethmoid sinus
F frontal lobe
FS frontal sinus
Ft intraorbital fat
FV fourth ventricle
G genu of corpus callosum
HI hippocampus
HP hard palate
IC internal carotid artery
ICo inferior concha
IJ internal jugular vein

IN external occipital
  protuberance
IO obliquus capitis inferior
IR inferior rectus
L lens
LF lateral fissure
LP lateral pterygoid
LSU lambdoidal suture
LV2 body (parietal horn) of
  lateral ventricle
LV3 posterior (occipital) horn
  of lateral ventricle

LV4 inferior (temporal) horn
  of lateral ventricle lateral
  ventricle
MA masseter
MAC mastoid air cells
ME medulla oblongata
MN1 head of mandible
MN2 ramus of mandible
MN3 body of mandible
MN4 mentis of mandible
MP medial pterygoid
MR medial rectus
MS maxillary sinus

NP nasopharynx
NS nasal septum
O occipital lobe
ON optic nerve
P parietal lobe
PF parietooccipital fissure
PG parotid gland
PI pituitary gland
PO pons
S splenium of corpus
  callosum
SCP semispinalis capitis
SMG submandibular gland

SR superior rectus
SS sphenoid sinus
SSS superior sagittal sinus
SVS superior vermian cistern
T temporal lobe
TE teeth
TG tongue
TL thalamus
TM temporalis
TS transverse sinus
TZ trapezius

14

PLATE 8. Slightly oblique, anterior part of right orbit, middle of left orbit, body of mandible, zygomatic bone: T1 MR image

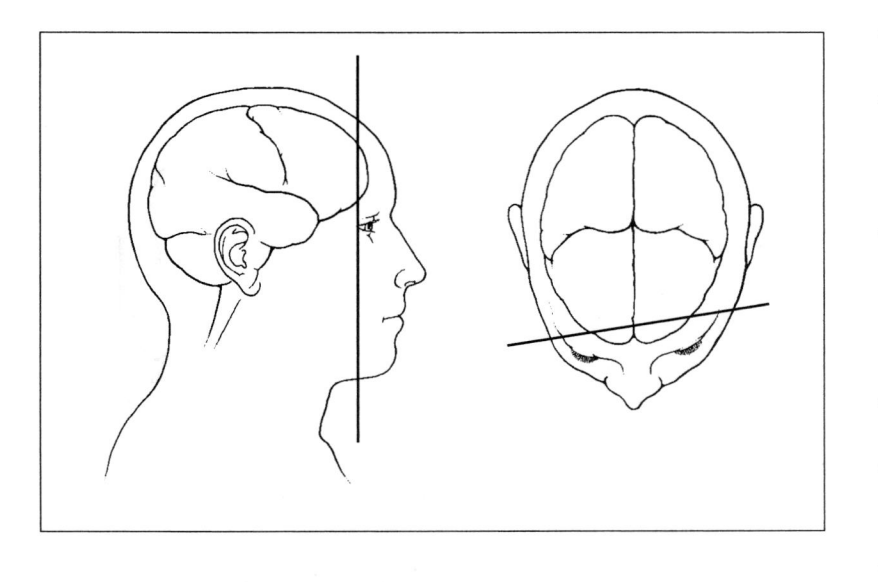

Note

- The **frontal lobes** (*F*) of the cerebrum exposed by a section through the **frontal bone** (*FB*) lie superior to the orbits.
- Extending inferiorly from the **superior sagittal sinus** (*SSS*), the **falx cerebri** (*FC*) attaches to the **crista galli** (*CG*) of the ethmoid bone. The **crista galli** (*CG*) extends inferiorly into the perpendicular plate of the ethmoid bone between the **ethmoid sinuses** (*ES*) which continues as the upper part of the **nasal septum** (*NS*).
- The lateral walls of the **ethmoid sinuses** (*ES*) form the medial walls of the orbit, whose contents on the right include the **eyeball** (*E*), and on the left, which is more posterior, the **optic nerve** (*ON*). Extraocular muscles, seen in both **A** and **B** include the **superior rectus** (*SR*), **superior oblique** (*SO*), **inferior rectus** (*IR*), and **lateral rectus** (*LR*). The **inferior oblique** (*IOB*) is seen in **A**. The **lacrimal gland** (*LG*) appears in the upper lateral quadrant of the orbit.
- The structures identified by *Co* are the **inferior and middle nasal conchae**. They lie on the lateral sides of the nasal cavity and are closely related to the **maxillary sinuses** (*MS*) lateral to them.
- Structures related to the oral cavity and floor of the mouth include the **tongue** (*TG*), **geniohyoid** (*GH*), **genioglossus** (*GG*), **mylohyoid** (*MH*), and **anterior belly of the digastric** (*DG*). Also seen is the **body of the mandible** (*MN3*).
- The **maxilla** (*MX*) forms part of the structure of the **hard palate** (*HP*), below which there is an **upper denture** (*DP*).

Clinical Notes

- The relationship between the nasal cavity and paranasal sinuses is optimally shown on coronal images. This image reveals that the nasal septum is slightly deviated from right to left.
- Only thin tables of bone separate the orbit, anterior cranial fossa, ethmoid sinus, sphenoid sinus, and nasal cavity. Fractures, penetration by sharp objects, or erosion by osteolytic cancerous growth can easily occur.
- A blow to the apex of the nose may cause a cribriform plate fracture leading to a meningeal laceration and resultant leakage of cerebrospinal fluid through the nasal passages (rhinorrhea).

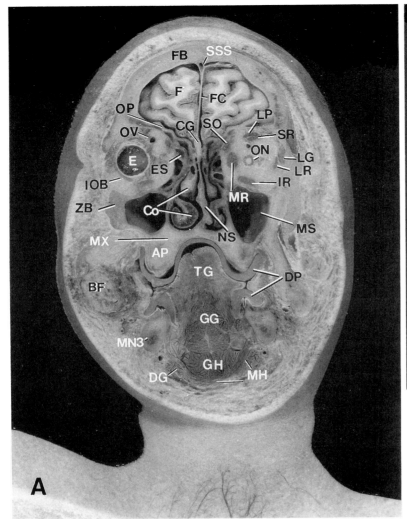

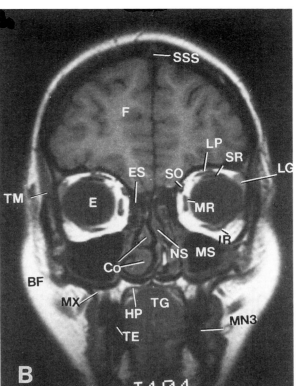

16

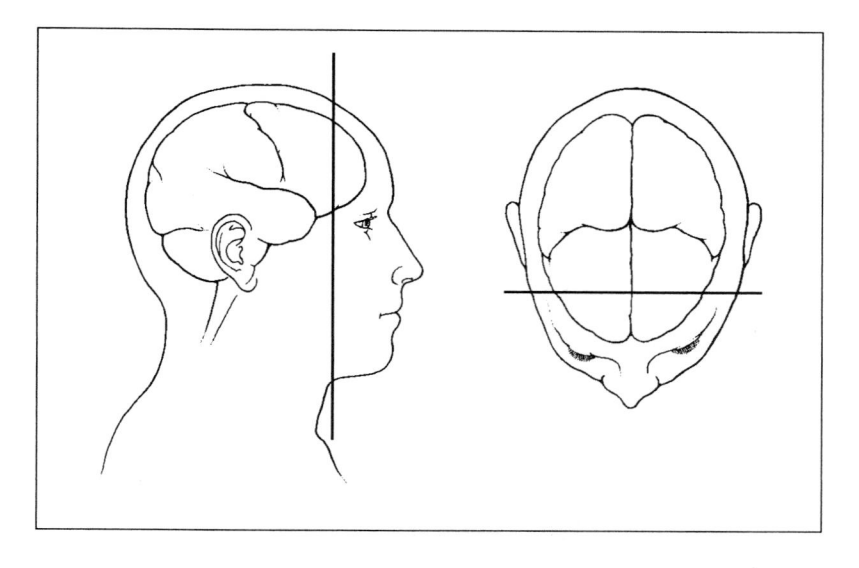

Note

- The **frontal lobes** (*F*) of the cerebrum are exposed by a slightly oblique section passing through the posterior part of the orbits.
- The perpendicular plate of the ethmoid bone is related on both sides to the **ethmoid sinuses** (*ES*), which themselves form the medial walls of the orbits. The orbital contents clearly seen here include the extraocular muscles described in plate 8, **intraorbital fat** (*Ft*) and the **optic nerve** (*ON*).
- To the lateral sides of the nasal septum lie the **inferior nasal concha** (*ICo*) and the **middle nasal concha** (*MC*) of the nasal cavity. The **optic nerve** (*ON*) emerges from the posterior part of the orbits. Inferior to the orbit on the right in **A** and left in **B** is the posterior wall of the **maxillary sinus** (*MS*). On the lateral side of this orbit is the **greater wing of the sphenoid bone** (*GW*).
- Two of the muscles of mastication, **temporalis** (*TM*) and **masseter** (*MA*), appear here.
- The **anterior (frontal) horn of the lateral ventricle** (*LV1*) is seen in **B**, which is slightly posterior to the plane in **A**.
- Structures related to the oral cavity and floor of the mouth include the **tongue** (*TG*), **mylohyoid** (*MH*), **hyoglossus** (*HG*), **lamina of thyroid cartilage** (*TY*), **epiglottis** (*EG*), and **body** (*MN3*) of the mandible.

Clinical Notes

- The appearance of compact bone compared to marrow is reviewed here using the **body of the mandible** (*MN3*) as an example. The number *1* points to the to compact bone, which gives a low-intensity signal and is black. The number *2* points to the marrow of the mandible, which gives a higher intensity signal and is brighter.
- The extent of sinus disease, with mucoperiosteal thickening and the presence of air fluid levels, is well seen on MR images. The adequacy of surgical decompression and the origin and invasion of neoplasms such as squamous cell carcinomas can be evaluated. However, fine bone detail of the sinuses is still best evaluated by CT scans.

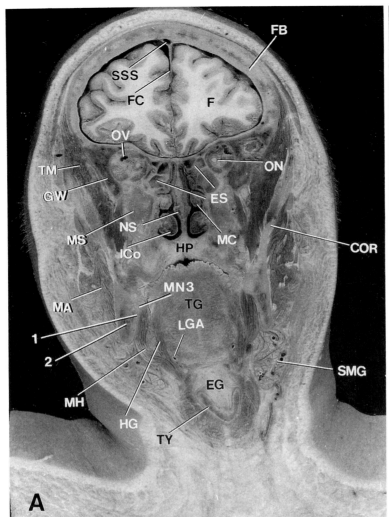

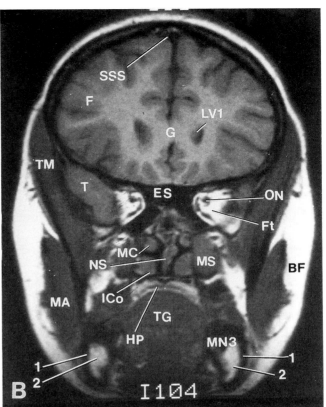

A

B I104

PLATE 10. Pituitary gland, sphenoid sinus, greater wing of sphenoid, and thyroid gland: T1 MR image

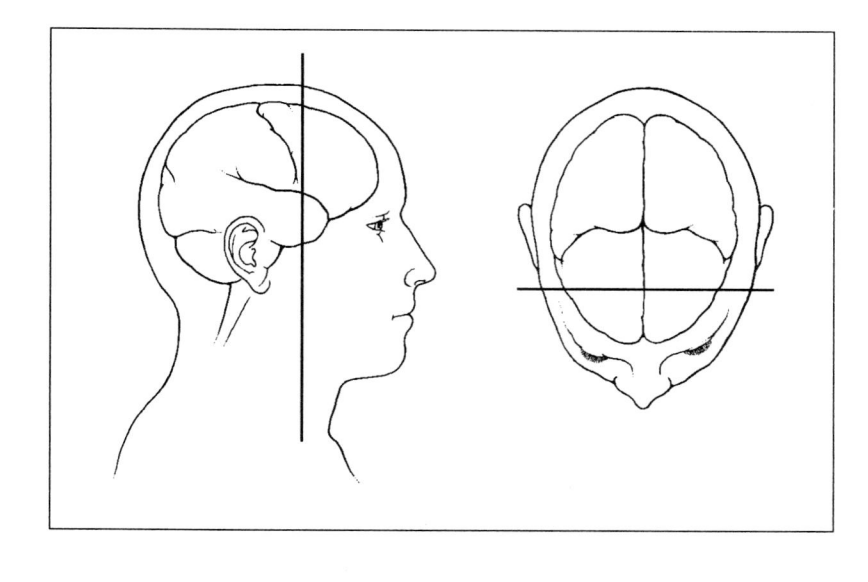

Note

- **B** is slightly anterior to **A**.
- The **frontal lobes** (*F*) and **temporal** (*T*) lobes of the cerebrum, separated by the **lateral or sylvian fissure** (*LF*) and the **insula** (*I*) are seen. The bodies of the left and right **lateral ventricles** (*LV*) and basal ganglia structures inferior to them appear here. These latter structures are the **putamen** (*PU*), **internal capsule** (*ICP*), and **head of the caudate nucleus** (*CN*), called collectively, the corpus striatum.
- Forming the roof of the **bodies of the lateral ventricles** (*LV2*) is the **body of the corpus callosum** (*B*), and separating the left from the right one is the **septum pellucidum** (*SP*).
- Medial to the temporal lobes, which rest on the **greater wing of the sphenoid bone** (*GW*), is the **cavernous sinus** (*CV*), containing the **internal carotid artery** (*IC*), which is cut twice as it forms the carotid siphon. Important nerves to the extraocular muscles and the ophthalmic division of the trigeminal, not clearly seen here, are on its lateral side. The **pituitary gland** (*PI*) occupies the hyophyseal fossa, which forms part of the roof of the **sphenoid sinus** (*SS*).
- The posterior part of the **optic chiasma** (*X*) lies just above the anterior lobe of the **pituitary gland** (*PI*).
- The **sphenoid sinus** (*SS*) lies superior to the **nasopharynx** (*NP*), which itself is between the left and right parapharyngeal regions related to the infratemporal region. Here, the principal muscular contents of the infratemporal region, the **lateral pterygoid** (*LP*) and **medial pterygoid** (*MP*), are seen. The **medial pterygoid** (*MP*) attaches to the medial side of the mandible on the lateral side of which attaches the **masseter muscle** (*MA*).
- In a direct line running inferiorly from the **nasopharynx** (*NP*) are the **soft palate** (*SPA*), **oropharynx** (*PH*), and **epiglottis** (*EG*). Note also the **larynx** (*LX*) and **trachea** (*Tr*). To the sides of the **trachea** (*Tr*) and the lower part of the **larynx** (*LX*) and its related cartilages are the left and right lobes of the **thyroid gland** (*TYG*).

Clinical Notes

- Size and position of the ventricles is critical in the diagnosis of neural pathology.
- Pituitary gland tumors may extend superiorly through the aperture of the diaphragma sellae and compress the optic chiasma.

*References **G** 4-81A and B, 7-131B; **N** 96; **RY** 64, 92*

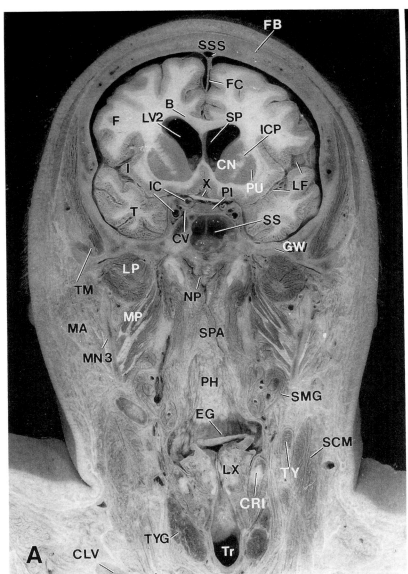

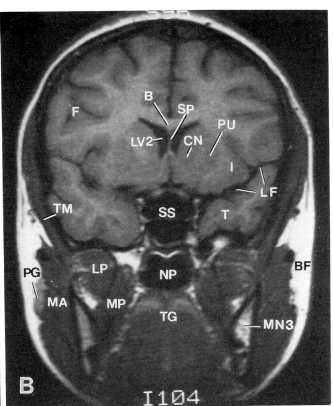

I104

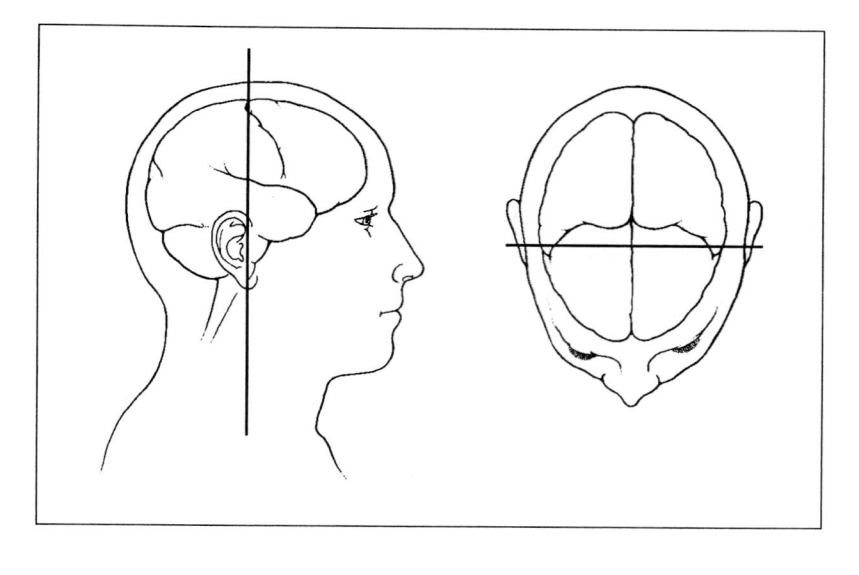

Note

- The **frontal** (*F*) and **temporal lobes** (*T*) of the cerebrum are separated by the **lateral or sylvian fissure** (*LF*) and the **insula** (*I*). The bodies of the left and right **lateral ventricles** (*LV2*) and between the left and right **thalami** (*TH*) the **third ventricle** (*TV*) are seen.
- Anterolateral to the **thalamus** (*TH*) is the **putamen** (*PU*), which lies deep to the cortex of the **insula** (*I*). Inferolateral to the **putamen** (*PU*) is the **temporal lobe** (*T*), containing the **inferior (temporal) horn of the lateral ventricle** (**LV4**), whose medial wall is formed in part by the **hippocampus** (*HI*).
- The **basilar artery** (*BA*) makes its appearance below the **pons** (*PO*) and is here just posterior to the **basioccipital bone** (*OB*) at this point. Lateral to the **pons** (*PO*) in **B** is the **trigeminal nerve** (*TN*).
- In a direct line running inferiorly from the **basiocciput** (*OB*) are the cervical vertebrae. The **first cervical vertebra (atlas)** (*CV1*) articulates with the occipital condyles at the **atlantooccipital joint** (*OJ*). Inferiorly, it articulates with the **second cervical vertebra (axis)** (*CV2*), at the **atlantoaxial joint** (*ATX*).
- Continuing inferiorly, the **pharynx** (*PH*), **esophagus** (*E*), and **trachea** (*Tr*) are seen. To both sides of the trachea are the **common carotid arteries** (*CC*).

Clinical Notes

- The venous sinuses are demonstrated noninvasively by MR imaging.
- Venous thrombosis can occur in hypercoagulable states, such as those found in the postpartum patient. The degree of venous invasion is important in planning resection of adjacent meningiomas.
- Cavernous sinus thrombosis is less common than superior sagittal sinus thrombosis, which itself is uncommon.
- The more posterior one goes, the more the basal ganglia (putamen, caudate nucleus) disappear and the thalamus is seen.

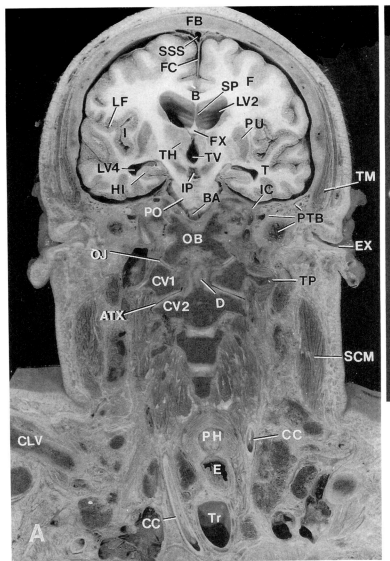

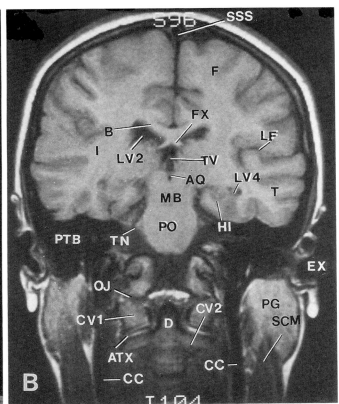

PLATE 12. Sigmoid sinus, fourth ventricle, mastoid process and mastoid air cells: T1 MR image

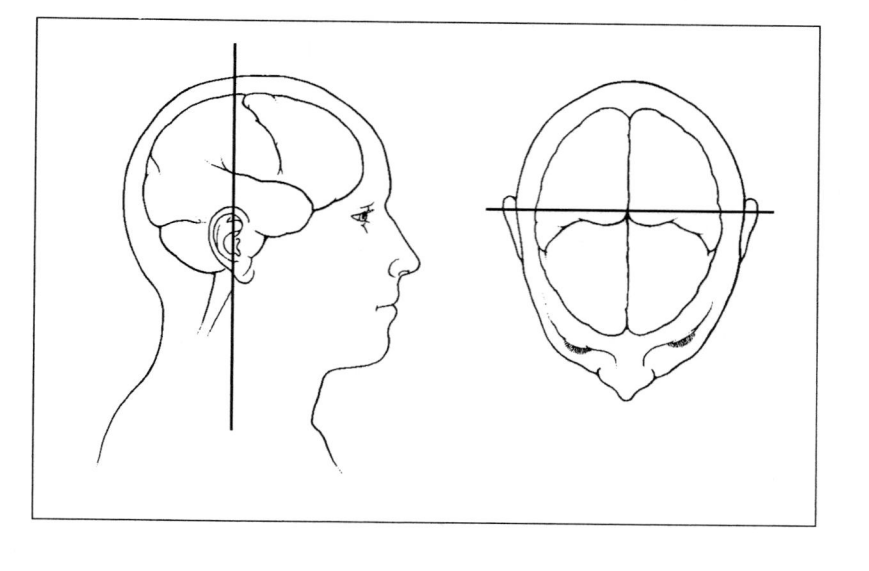

Note

- The **parietal** (*P*) and **temporal** (*T*) lobes of the cerebrum are separated by the lateral or sylvian fissure (unlabeled). The posterior part of the **bodies of the left and right lateral ventricles** (*LV2*) appear at the atrium (trigone) of the lateral ventricles.
- Inferior to the splenium is the **epithalamus**, or **pineal body** (*EP*), overhanging a piece of the collicular portion of the **mesencephalon (midbrain)** (*MB*).
- The cerebral lobes are separated from the **cerebellum** (*CE*) by the **tentorium cerebelli** (*TC*). In the cerebellar midline is the **fourth ventricle** (*FV*), outlined superiorly by the **superior cerebellar peduncle (brachium conjunctivum)** (*BC*) and inferiorly by the **inferior cerebellar peduncle (restiform body)** (*RB*). The floor of this ventricle is formed by the caudal part of the pons and the cranial part of the medulla and is visible through the opening made by sectioning.
- To the lateral sides of the cerebellum is the mastoid portion of the temporal bone containing the **mastoid air cells** (*MAC*) and a part of the **sigmoid sinus** (*SG*).
- Caudal to the region of the **fourth ventricle** (*FV*), the spinal canal begins at the **foramen magnum** (*white dots*) and is lined by **dura mater** (*DM*). The **occipital bone** (*OB*) and the **anterior arch of the first cervical vertebra** (*AA*), above which lies the **vertebral artery** (*VA*), are also seen.
- More caudally and centrally, a part of the **cervical spinal cord** (*C*) has been sectioned, as have **vertebral bodies** (*VB*) and **disks** (*DK*).
- Lateral to the vertebra, portions of the paravertebral muscles are seen. Lateral to them is the **sterno-cleidomastoid** (*SCM*).

Clinical Notes

- Normal mastoid air cells are not delineated because of the low signal (black) from air and bone.
- The choroid plexus found in all the ventricles produces cerebrospinal fluid. Often it is incidentally calcified and appears as a radiopacity on plain radiographs and on CT scans.
- The atrium of the lateral ventricle (junction of body, posterior, and inferior (temporal) horn of lateral ventricles) defines lobar anatomy. Above the atrium is the parietal lobe, inferior to it is the temporal lobe, and posterior to it is the occipital lobe.

References G *7-33;* **N** *102, 109;* **RY** *112, 159, 160*

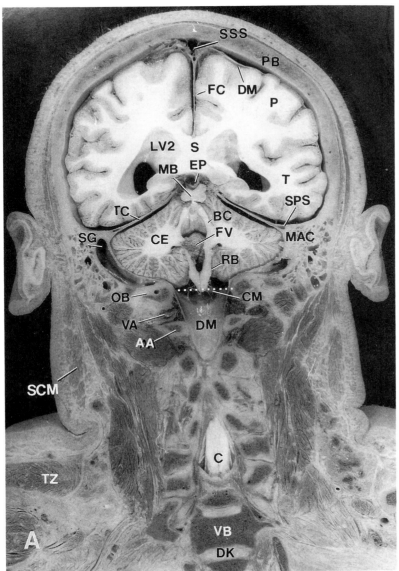

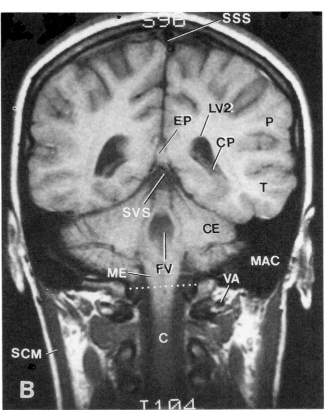

Chapter I. Head and Neck
Part II. Coronal Sections

25

PLATE 13. Transverse sinus, superior sagittal sinus, inferior sagittal sinus, suboccipital triangle, spine of CV2: T1 MR image

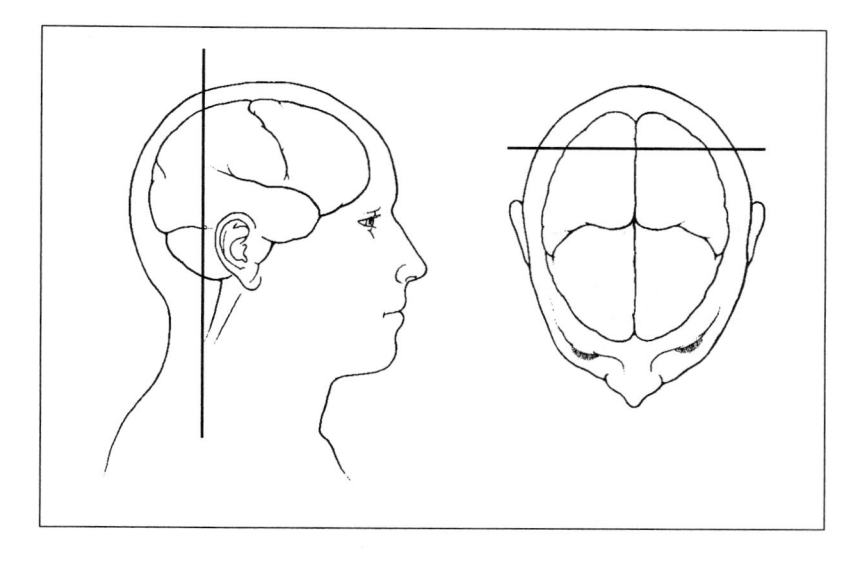

Note

- The **occipital lobe** (*O*) of the cerebrum contains the **posterior (occipital) horn of the lateral ventricle** (*LV3*).
- The **falx cerebri** (*FC*), separating the left and right parietal lobes of the cerebrum, is continuous with the **tentorium cerebelli** (*TC*). At its upper end, the falx helps to form the **superior sagittal sinus** (*SSS*), and at its lower end, it helps to form the **inferior sagittal sinus** (*ISS*). The **transverse sinuses** (*TS*) close to their terminations in the sigmoid sinuses are seen at the lateral edges of the **tentorium cerebelli** (*TC*).
- Inferior to the **vermis of the cerebellum** (*VC*) is the expanded part of the subarachnoid space known as the **cisterna magna (cerebellomedullary cistern)** (*CM*).
- Just inferior to the portion of the **occipital bone** (*OB*) seen here, is the **suboccipital triangle** (*SOT*) region, a key localizing feature of which is the **spine of the second cervical vertebra** (*CV2*).
- Lateral to the vertebra, portions of the deep back muscles are seen and far laterally, the **sternocleidomastoid** (*SCM*).

Clinical Notes

- The cerebellar vermis preferentially atrophies with alcohol abuse and with chronic dilantin use. The clinical significance of this is unclear.

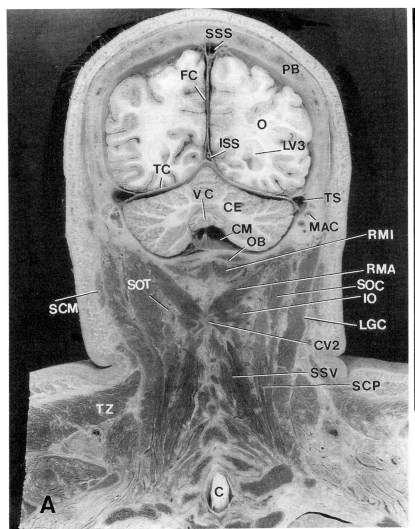

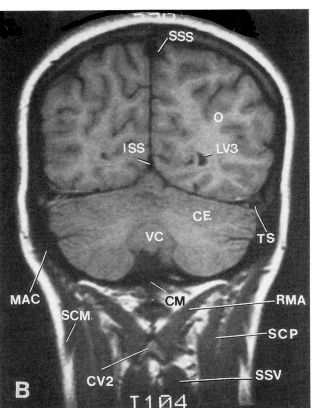

KEY

C cervical spinal cord
CE cerebellum
CM cisterna magna
CV2 spine, CV2

FC falx cerebri
IO obliquus capitis inferior
ISS inferior sagittal sinus
LGC longissimus capitis

LV3 posterior (occipital) horn, lateral ventricle
MAC mastoid air cells
O occipital lobe
OB occipital bone

PB parietal bone
RMA rectus capitis major
RMI rectus capitis minor
SCM sternocleidomastoid
SCP semispinalis capitis

SOC obliquus capitis superior
SOT suboccipital triangle
SSS superior sagittal sinus
SSV semispinalis cervicis
TC tentorium cerebelli

TS transverse sinus
TZ trapezius
VC vermis of cerebellum

PLATE 14. Sequential T1 MR coronal image overview of the head

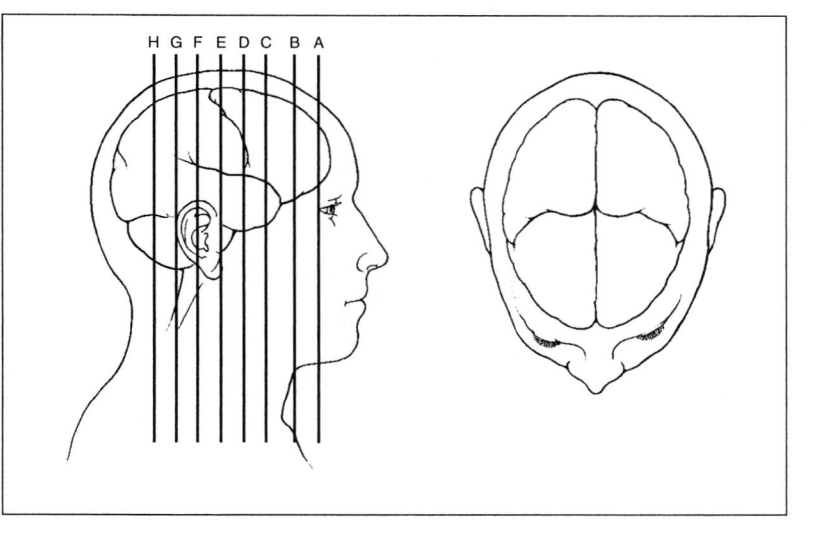

Note

As mentioned in the introduction and notes for the first review sequence (Plate 7), the analysis of sequential images shows how sectional anatomy can be used to learn structural relationships. Cross-references between coronal, sagittal, and transaxial sections and images will enable the student to better conceptualize three-dimensional structure and relationships. As one example, the plate below, with images oriented from anterior **A** to posterior **H**, show the lateral ventricles through most of their extent. The changing form of these structures at different levels can profitably be compared to sagittal and transaxial views of the head (as for example this plate with Plate 7).

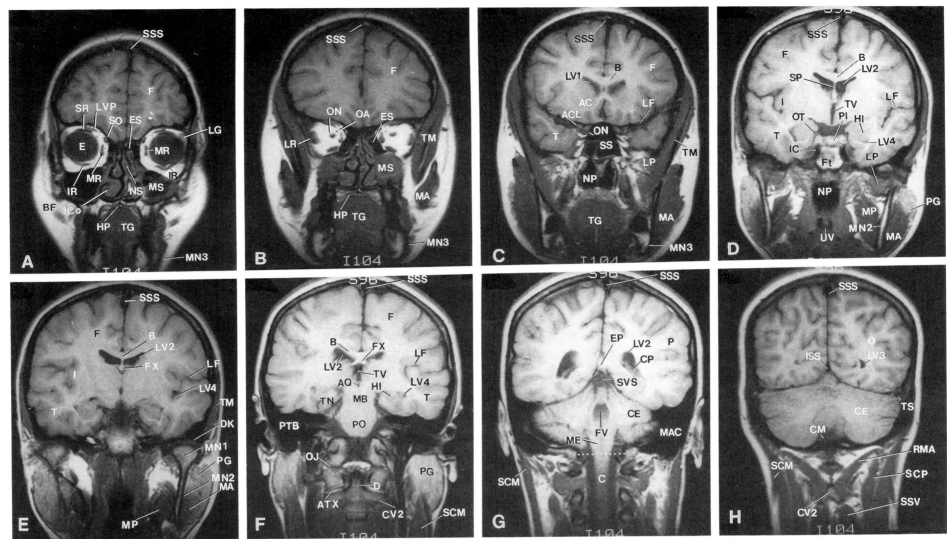

KEY

KEY

AC anterior commissure
ACL anterior clinoid process
AQ cerebral aqueduct
ATX atlantoaxial joint
B body of corpus callosum
BF buccal fat
C cervical spinal cord
CE cerebellum
CM cisterna magna
CP choroid plexus
CV2 (*F*) transverse process, CV2
CV2 (*H*) spine, CV2

D dens (odontoid process)
DK disk of temporomandibular joint
E eyeball
EP pineal gland
ES ethmoid sinus
F frontal lobe
Ft marrow fat in clivus
FV fourth ventricle
FX fornix
HI hippocampus
HP hard palate
I insula
IC internal carotid

ICo inferior nasal concha
IR inferior rectus
ISS inferior sagittal sinus
LF lateral fissure
LG lacrimal gland
LP lateral pterygoid
LR lateral rectus
LV1 anterior (frontal) horn, lateral ventricle
LV2 body (parietal horn), lateral ventricle
LV3 posterior (occipital) horn, lateral ventricle

LV4 inferior (temporal) horn, lateral ventricle
LVP levator palpebrae
MA masseter
MAC mastoid air cells
MB mesencephalon
ME medulla oblongata
MN1 head of mandible
MN2 ramus of mandible
MN3 body of mandible
MP medial pterygoid
MR medial rectus
MS maxillary sinus
NP nasopharynx

NS nasal septum
OA ophthalmic artery
OJ atlanto-occipital joint
ON optic nerve
OT optic tract
P parietal lobe
PG parotid gland
PI pituitary gland
PO pons
PTB petrous temporal bone
RMA rectus capitis major
SCM sternocleidomastoid
SCP semispinalis capitis
SO superior oblique

SP septum pellucidum
SR superior rectus
SS sphenoid sinus
SSS superior sagittal sinus
SSV semispinalis cervicis
SVS superior vermian cistern
T temporal lobe
TG tongue
TM temporalis
TN trigeminal nerve
TS transverse sinus
TV third ventricle
UV uvula

28

PLATE 15. Centrum semiovale, ascending and descending parts of the superior sagittal sinus: T1 MR image

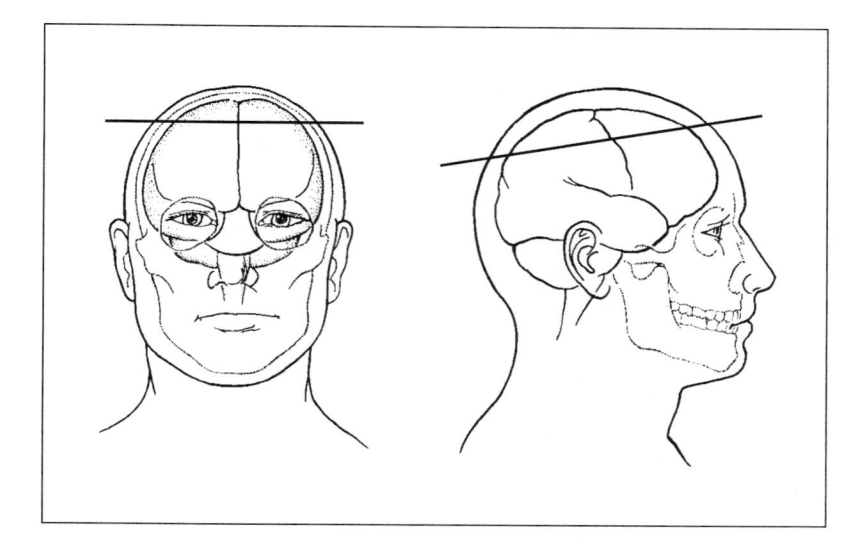

Note

- **Frontal** (*F*), **parietal** (*P*), and **occipital** (*O*) lobes of the cerebrum are here surrounded by **frontal** (*FB*) and **occipital** (*OB*) calvarial bones.
- The **falx cerebri** (*FC*) lies in the superior sagittal fissure, which separates left and right cerebral hemispheres.
- The gyri of the cerebrum are rimmed by more darkly shaded gray matter of the **cerebral cortex** (*CX*) surrounding the white matter. The central portion of the white matter defines the **centrum semiovale** (*CSO*).
- The **superior sagittal sinus** (*SSS*) is sectioned twice as it ascends anteriorly and descends posteriorly.
- The **fat of the scalp** (*4*) and the **diplöe** (*2*) in **B** show an intermediate signal (white) and stand out in strong contrast to the **compact bone of the inner and outer tables of the calvaria** (*1, 3*).

Clinical Notes

- Magnetic resonance (MR) imaging is the most sensitive technique for visualizing intracerebral pathology.
- Clinically, T1 images are used to detect the bright signal of subarachnoid hemorrhage.

References G 4-64, 7-15; *RY 85, 114*

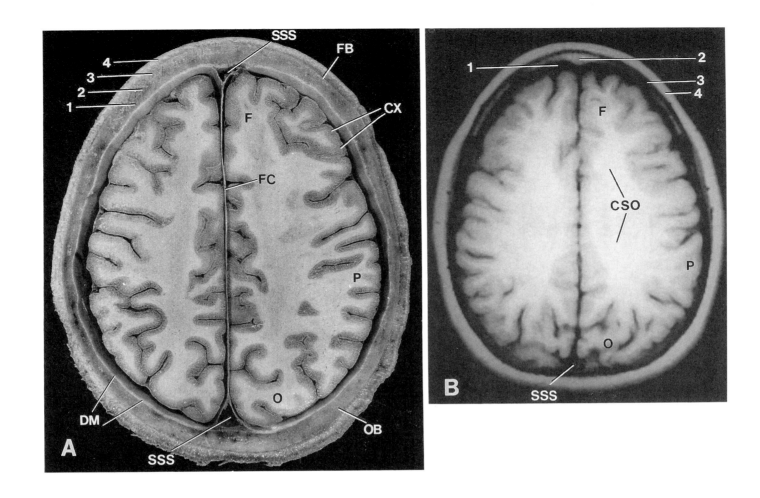

PLATE 16. Genu, body, and splenium of corpus callosum: T1 MR image

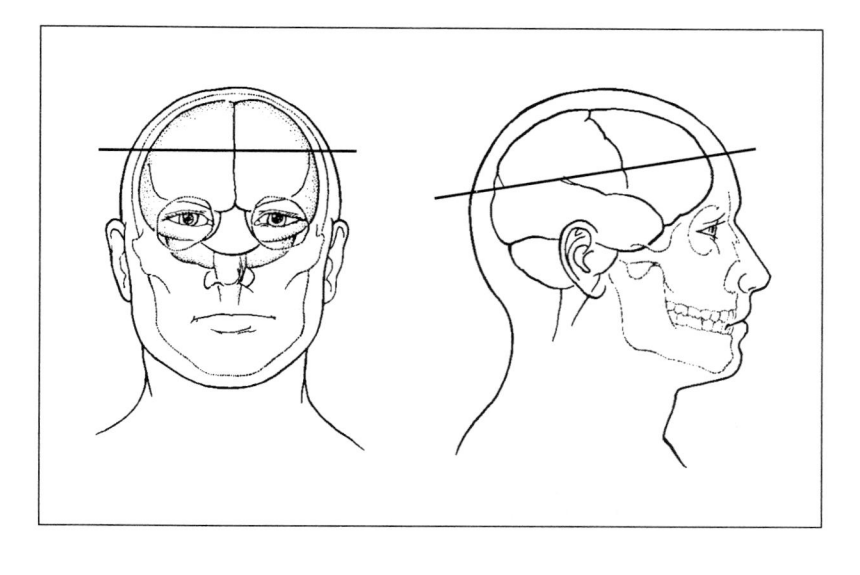

Note

- **B** is slightly inferior to **A**.
- **Frontal** (*F*), **parietal** (*P*), and **occipital** (*O*) lobes of the cerebrum are surrounded by **frontal** (*FB*), **parietal** (*PB*), and **occipital** (*OB*) calvarial bone.
- The **falx cerebri** (*FC*) lies in the **superior sagittal fissure** (*SF*) separating the two frontal lobes anteriorly and the occipital lobes posteriorly.
- The gyri of the cerebrum are rimmed by darker-shaded **cerebral cortex (gray matter)** (*CX*) surrounding white matter.
- The **superior sagittal sinus** (*SSS*) is sectioned as it descends posteriorly toward the confluence of sinuses (Plate 17).
- The **genu** (*G*), **body** (*B*) and **splenium** (*S*), of the corpus callosum form the roof of the **anterior (frontal) horn, body, and posterior (occipital) horn** of the **lateral ventricles** (*LV1, LV2, LV3*). Part of the **choroid plexus** (*CP*) appears in the ventricles. The **caudate nucleus** labeled at its **body** (*CNb*) and **tail** (*CNt*) helps form the ventricular wall. The **anterior cerebral artery** (*ACA*) lies anterior to the **genu** (*G*).
- The **lateral ventricles** are surrounded by **periventricular white matter** (*PV*).
- The **superior sagittal sinus** (*SSS*) is formed by the **dura mater** (*DM*).
- The **optic radiation** (*OR*) coursing to the visual cortex is seen in the **occipital** (*O*) **lobe**.
- The **central sulcus** (*CS*) of the cerebrum is accentuated by the dark signal of cerebrospinal fluid (CSF) in **B**.

Clinical Notes

- Periventricular white matter tract lesions occurring in multiple sclerosis and other demyelinating diseases are well seen in MR images.

*References **G** 7-30; **N** 102; **RY** 114, 115*

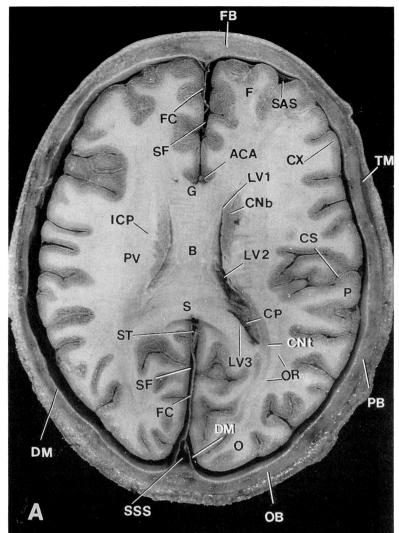

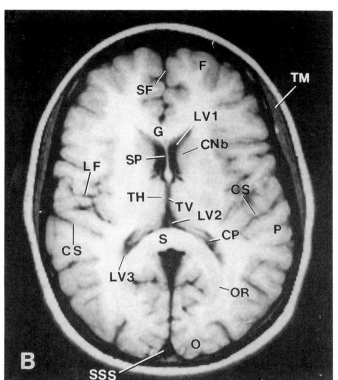

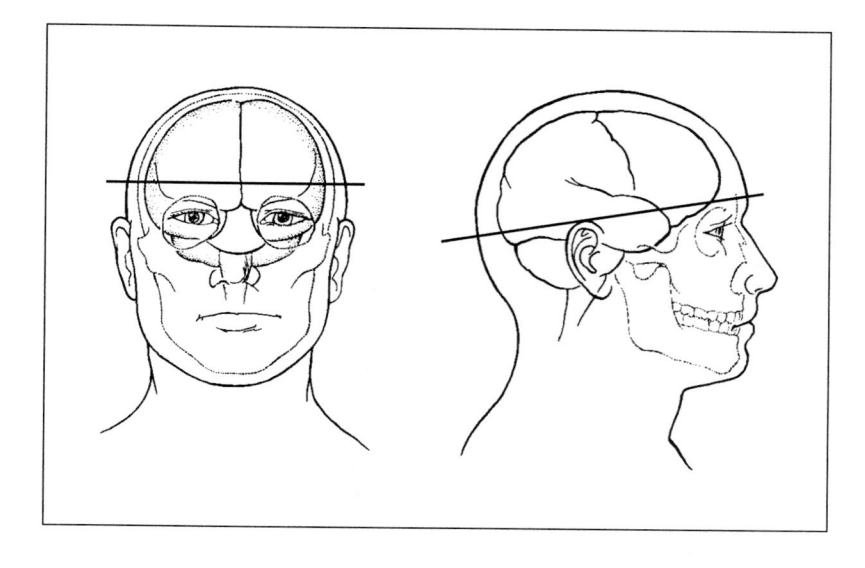

Note

- **Frontal** (*F*), **temporal** (*T*), and **occipital** (*O*) lobes of the cerebrum are surrounded by **frontal** (*FB*), **parietal** (*PB*), **temporal** (*TB*), and **occipital** (*OB*) bones.
- The **superior sagittal fissure** (*SF*) separates the **frontal lobes** (*F*) and is here delimited posteriorly by the **anterior commissure** (*ACM*) anterior to the **third ventricle** (*TV*). The **frontal** (*F*) and **temporal** (*T*) lobes are separated by the **lateral or sylvian fissure** (*LF*).
- The important **middle cerebral artery** (*MCA*) is difficult to see in this section, but it appears at several points in its course in the **lateral fissure** (*LF*).
- Centrally, brainstem and basal ganglia structures appear. The head of the **caudate nucleus** (*CNh*) lies anterior to the **anterior commissure** (*ACM*). Posterior to it is the **optic tract** (*OTR*), passing into the **lateral geniculate body** (*LGE*), which itself lies lateral to the **medial geniculate body** (*MG*) and medial to the **hippocampus** (*HI*).
- The **internal capsule** (*ICP*) is seen just above its entrance into the cerebral peduncles of the mesencephalon.
- The **transverse sinus** (*TS*) is seen near to where it leaves the **confluence of sinuses (torcular herophilii)** (*CF*) lying posterior to the **cerebellum** (*CE*).

Clinical Notes

- Cisterns of the brain represent expansions of the CSF spaces. They are continuous with one another and are named somewhat arbitrarily, based on surrounding structures.

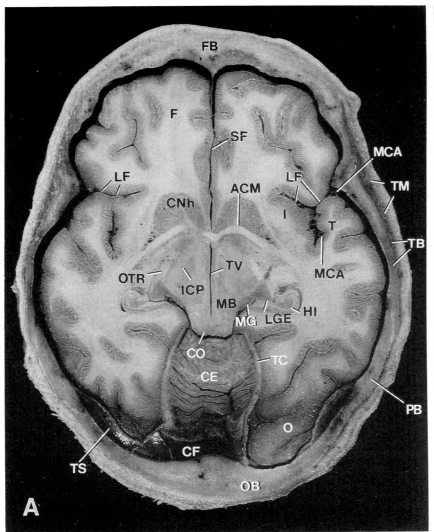

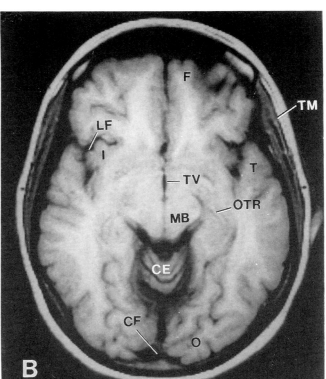

ACM anterior commissure	**CO** inferior colliculus	**ICP** internal capsule	**MG** medial geniculate body	**SF** superior sagittal fissure	**TS** transverse sinus
CE cerebellum	**F** frontal lobe	**LF** lateral fissure	**O** occipital lobe	**T** temporal lobe	**TV** third ventricle
CF confluence of sinuses	**FB** frontal bone	**LGE** lateral geniculate body	**OB** occipital bone	**TB** temporal bone	
CNh caudate nucleus (head)	**HI** hippocampus	**MB** mesencephalon	**OTR** optic tract	**TC** tentorium cerebelli	
	I insula	**MCA** middle cerebral artery	**PB** parietal bone	**TM** temporalis muscle	

PLATE 18. Eyeball, petrous temporal bone, tips of temporal lobes, pons: T1 MR image

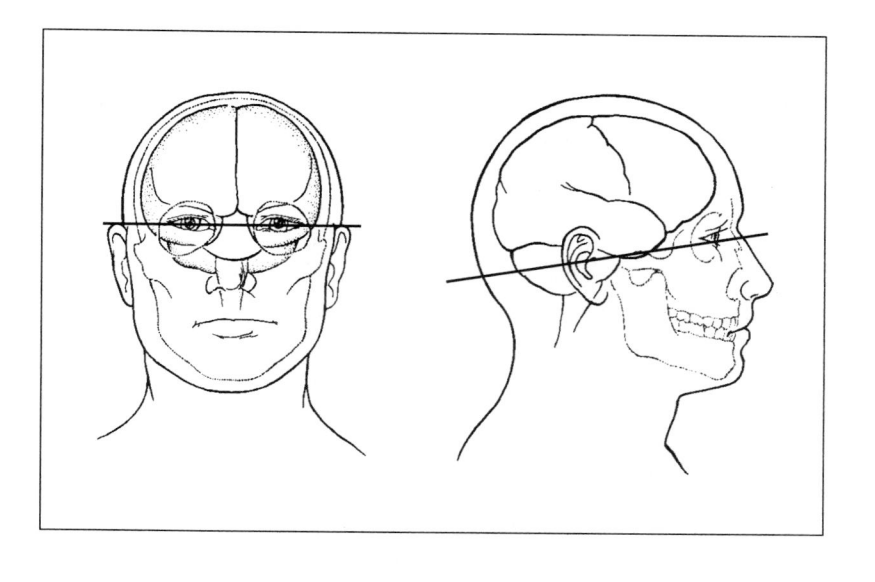

Note

- The **temporal** (*T*) lobe of the cerebrum occupies the middle cranial fossa. It is delimited anteriorly by the **greater wing of the sphenoid bone** (*GW*), laterally by the **squamous temporal bone** (*SQ*), inferiorly by the **petrous temporal bone** (*PTB*), and medially by midline structures described below.
- The orbits appear anteriorly and are marked by the **eyeball** (*E*), **lens** (*L*), **optic nerves** (*ON*) converging at right angles to one another, much **intraorbital fat** (*Ft*), and two of the extraocular muscles, **lateral rectus** (*LR*) and **medial rectus** (*MR*).
- The **ethmoid sinuses** (*ES*) lie between the orbits and anterior to the more centrally located **sphenoid sinus** (*SS*), which is related anteriorly to the **pituitary gland** (*PI*). On both sides of the pituitary lie the **cavernous sinuses** (*CV*) through which courses the **internal carotid artery** (*IC*).
- In the posterior cranial fossa behind the **clivus** (*CL*) and **petrous temporal bone** (*PTB*), and delimited posteriorly by the **occipital bone** (*OB*) lie the **pons** (*PO*) and to the **vermis** (*VC*) and **lateral lobe** (*LC*) of the cerebellum.
- The **sigmoid sinus** (*SG*) lies posterior to the petrous temporal bone.
- The **basilar artery** (*BA*) passes anterior to the pons. Seen here also is the more cranial part of the **fourth ventricle** (*FV*).
- The **trigeminal nerve** (*TN*) passes from the pons into the **cavernous sinus** (*CV*).

Clinical Notes

- Obstruction of the internal carotid artery can be diagnosed by MR imaging because of the difference in signal between clotted (light gray) and free-flowing blood (black).
- Because of its sensitivity, MR imaging is the modality of choice in evaluating temporal lobe lesions.
- MR imaging is also optimal for evaluation of the cerebrum, cerebellum, and brainstem in the posterior cranial fossa since it eliminates bone artifacts present with CT scans. It is useful in revealing brainstem infarctions, neoplasms, and demyelinating diseases such as multiple sclerosis.

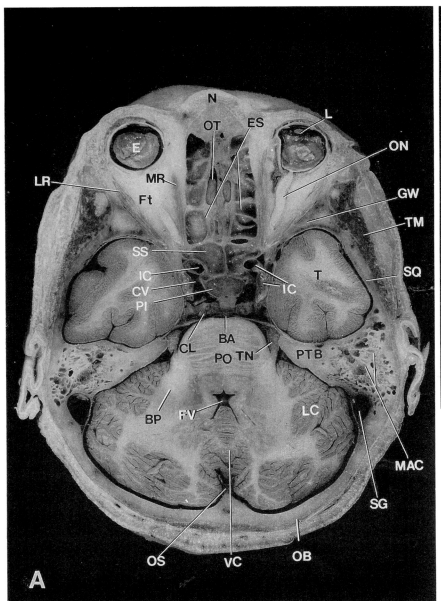

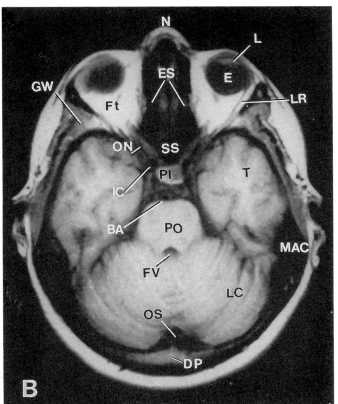

KEY _____

BA basilar artery
BP middle cerebellar
 peduncle
CL clivus
CV cavernous sinus

DP diplöe
E eyeball
ES ethmoid sinus
Ft intraorbital fat
FV fourth ventricle
GW greater wing of sphenoid

IC internal carotid artery
L lens
LC lateral lobe of cerebellum
LR lateral rectus
MAC mastoid air cells
MR medial rectus

N bridge of nose
OB occipital bone
ON optic nerve
OS occipital sinus
OT olfactory tract
PI pituitary gland

PO pons
PTB petrous temporal bone
SG sigmoid sinus
SQ squamous temporal bone
SS sphenoid sinus
T temporal lobe

TM temporalis muscle
TN trigeminal nerve
VC vermis of cerebellum

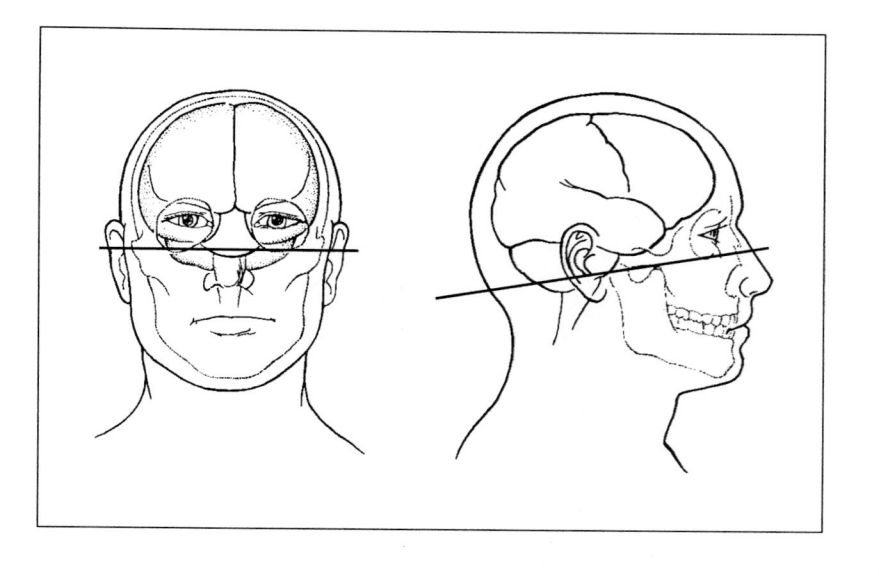

Note

- The surroundings of deeper structures at this level include the **upper nose** (*N*), the inferior part of the orbital cavity containing **intraorbital fat** (*Ft*), the **zygomatic bone** (*ZB*), part of the ear and the **external auditory meatus** (*EX*), and posteriorly, overlaid by deep and superficial back muscles, the **occipital bone** (*OB2*).
- Components of the nasal septum include anteriorly the **cartilaginous part** (*CR*) and a bony part, the **vomer** (*V*). To both sides of the septum lie the **nasal cavities** (*NC*), within which are the **inferior nasal concha** (*ICo*) and the **inferior meatus** (*IM*).
- To the lateral side of the nasal cavity appears the **maxillary sinus** (*MS*), whose roof can be seen to closely approximate the orbit above it. Lateral to this sinus, the **zygomatic bone** (*ZB*) and **zygomatic arch** (*ZA*) appear. Deep to the arch lies the **temporalis muscle** (*TM*), and medial to this muscle is the **lateral pterygoid** (*LP*) muscle. The latter crosses the infratemporal region to insert into the neck of the mandible and disk of the temporomandibular joint.
- The **basioccipital bone** (*OB1*) lies behind the sphenoid bone and to its lateral side can be seen the **auditory tube** (*AT*) and the **internal carotid artery** (*IC*) in the carotid canal.
- Posterior to the **internal carotid artery** (*IC*) on the left, lies the **sigmoid sinus** (*SG*), here just superior to the jugular foramen, which is out of the plane of section.
- The two **vertebral arteries** (*VA*) straddle the **medulla** (*ME*), posterior to which is the lower part of the **fourth ventricle** (*FV*).
- The inferior border of the **basiocciput** (*OB1*) forms the anterior portion of the foramen magnum.

Clinical Notes

- In **A**, the relationships that explain the spread of infection from the nasopharynx into the auditory tube, middle ear, and mastoid air cells can be seen.

References **G** *7-128 A,B;* **N** *116;* **RY** *42*

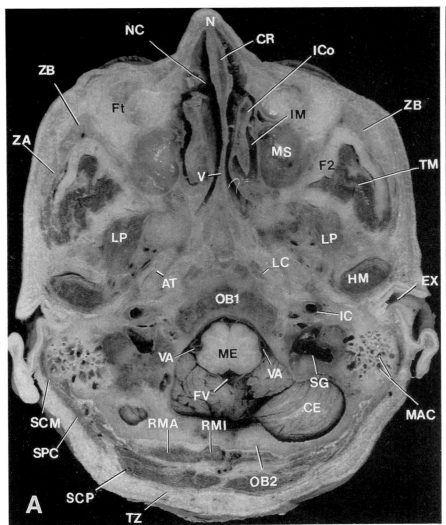

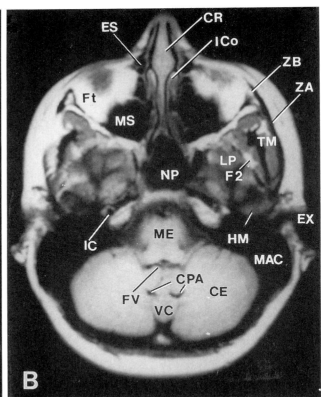

PLATE 20. Inferior nasal concha, lower maxillary sinus, odontoid process, and vertebral groove on atlas: T1 MR image

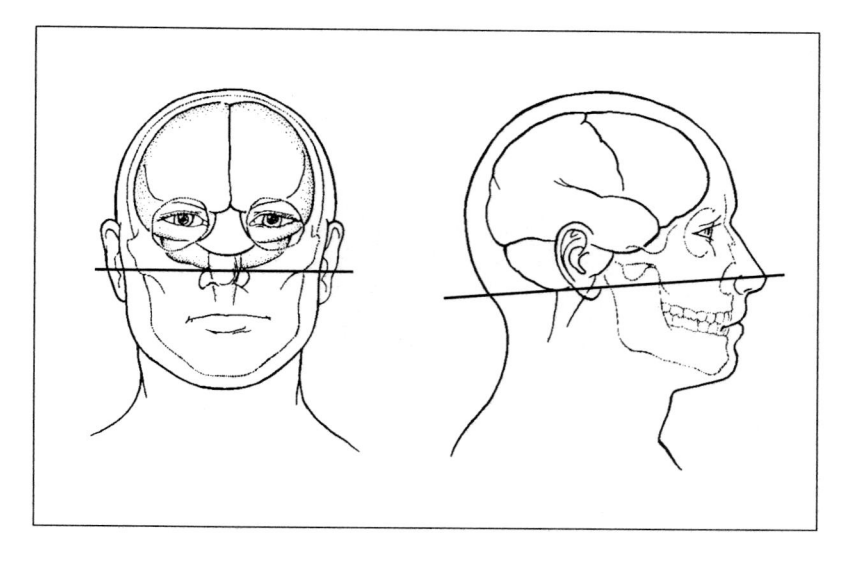

Note

- The surroundings of deeper structures at this level include the **middle nose** (*N*), the skin over **buccal fat** (*BF*), **maxillary bone** (*MX*), **temporalis muscle** (*TM*), **mandibular ramus** (*MR*), **parotid gland** (*PG*), and, behind it, part of the **external ear** (*EE*). Overlaid with deep and superficial muscles of the back of the neck is the **posterior arch of the atlas** (*PA*).
- Components of the nasal septum include anteriorly the **cartilaginous part** (*CR*) and a bony part, the **vomer** (*V*). To both sides of the septum lie the **nasal cavities** (*NC*), within which are the **inferior nasal concha** (*ICo*) and the **inferior meatus** (*IM*).
- To the sides of the nasal cavity is the **maxillary sinus** (*MS*), whose roof forms the inferior aspect of the orbit. The posterior wall of this sinus is mostly formed by the **maxillary bone** (*MX*).
- The **mandibular nerve** (*MNV*) lies between the medial pterygoid (*MP*) and **lateral pterygoid** (*LP*) muscles.
- The posterior part of the **nasal cavities** (*NC*) are continuous with the **nasopharynx** (*NP*), on whose roof are the **pharyngeal tonsils** (*PTO*).
- Posterior to the **nasopharynx** (*NP*) is the **anterior arch** (*AA*) of the **first cervical vertebra** (*CV1*). The **dens or odontoid process** (*D*) of CV2 articulates with its posterior aspect and lies just anterior to the **cervical spinal cord** (*C*).
- The **vertebral arteries** (*VA*) are here sectioned in their longitudinal courses in the vertebral arterial groove of the transverse process of CV1. Lateral to this lie the **internal carotid artery** (*IC*), **internal jugular vein** (*IJ*), and the **parotid gland** (*PG*).

Clinical Notes

- The soft tissue planes of the nasopharynx as seen in this MR image are used in the evaluation of nasopharyngeal masses.

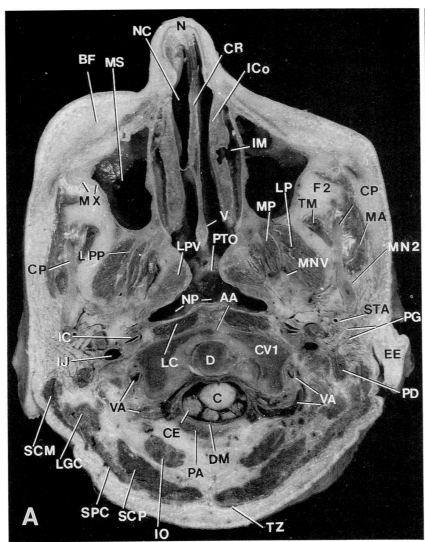

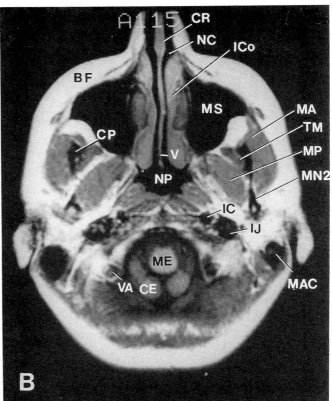

PLATE 21. CV2: upper region of alveolar processes of maxilla, soft palate, and spine of the second cervical vertebra: T1 MR image

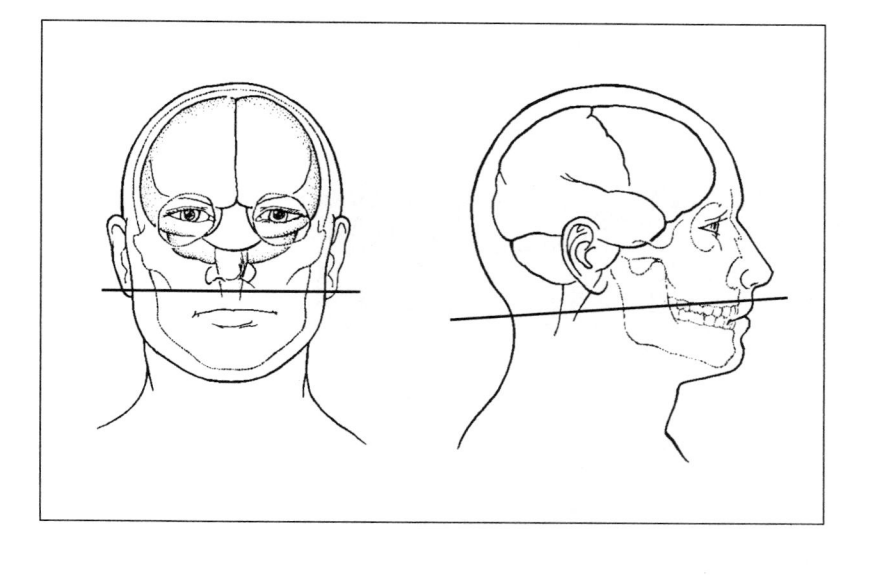

Note

- **B** is slightly higher than **A**.
- The surroundings of deeper structures at this level include the **upper lip** (*UL*), skin over the **buccal fat** (*BF*), and the **mandibular ramus** (*MN2*), covered laterally by the **masseter muscle** (*MA*) in front of the **parotid gland** (*PG*). Overlaid with deep and superficial muscles of the back of the neck, the **spine** (*SI*) and **lamina** (*LM*) of the **second cervical vertebra** (*CV2*).
- The alveolar process of the **maxillary arch** (*MX*) with **roots of maxillary teeth** (*MT*) embedded in it lies between the **vestibule** (*VM*) and **oral cavity** (*OC*).
- Just lateral to the **maxillary arch** (*MX*) lies the **buccinator muscle** (*BC*) following its course to the **pterygomandibular raphe** (*PR*), which also serves as an anterior attachment of the **superior pharyngeal constrictor** (*S*), forming the wall of the upper part of the **oropharynx** (*PH*).
- Posterior to the **pharynx** (*PH*) lies the lower part of the odontoid process of the **second cervical vertebra** (*CV2*). The **vertebral artery** (*VA*) is in the foramen transversarium of the transverse process on the right.
- Lateral to the **transverse process of CV2** (*TP*), labeled on its anterior tubercle, are the **internal carotid artery** (*IC*), **internal jugular vein** (*IJ*), and the **parotid gland** (*PG*).
- Within the spinal canal is the **cervical spinal cord** (*C*), surrounded by **spinal dura mater** (*DM*) and the **subarachnoid space** (*SAS*).
- The **mandibular ramus** (*MN2*) lies between the **medial pterygoid** (*MP*) medially and the **masseter** (*MA*) laterally.

Clinical Notes

- The root of the tongue is a common site for squamous cell cancer.

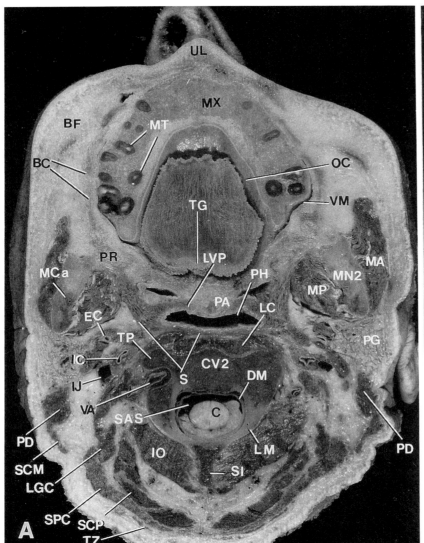

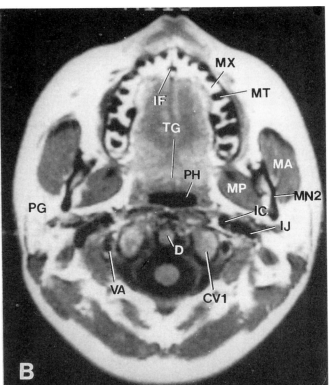

PLATE 22. CV2: upper dental arch, uvula, and body and spine of second cervical vertebra: T1 MR image

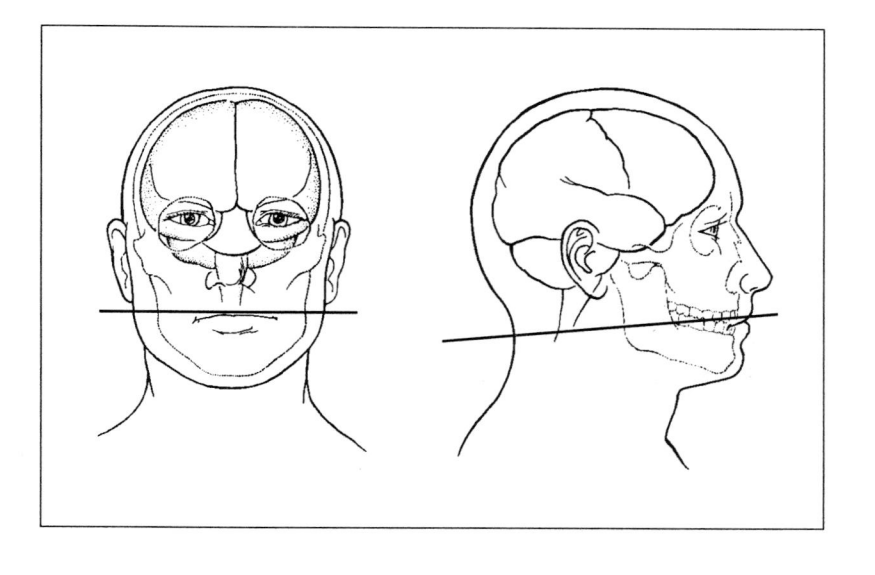

Note

- The surroundings of deeper structures at this level include the **upper lip** (*UL*), skin over the **buccal fat** (*BF*), **mandibular ramus** (*MN2*), and **masseter muscle** (*MA*), and the **spine** (*SI*) and **lamina** (*LM*) of the **second cervical vertebra** (*CV2*), overlaid with deep and superficial muscles of the back of the neck. (See also C and F of Plate 23, which are very close to this plane of section).
- Anteriorly, the dental arch, containing the maxillary **incisor** (*I*), **canine** (*CNT*), **premolar** (*PM*), and molar teeth, separates the **vestibule** (*VM*) and **oral cavity** (*OC*). The course of the **genioglossus** (*GG*) in the **tongue** (*TG*) is seen. Protruding inferiorly from the nasopharynx into the **oropharynx** (*PH*) near the root of the tongue is the **uvula** (*UV*).
- Posterior to the **oropharynx** (*PH*) lie the prevertebral muscles **longus colli** (*LCo*) and **longus capitis** (*LC*) on the anterior surface of the **second cervical vertebral body** (*CV2*). The **vertebral arteries** (*VA*) appear bilaterally in the transverse foramina. Lateral to this is the **internal carotid artery** (*IC*), **internal jugular vein** (*IJ*), and the **parotid gland** (*PG*). On the left, the **internal carotid artery** (*IC*) is seen posterior to the **external carotid artery** (*EC*).
- Within the spinal canal is the **cervical spinal cord** (*C*), surrounded by **spinal dura mater** (*DM*) and the subarachnoid space (unlabeled).
- The **mandibular ramus** (*MN2*) lies between the **medial pterygoid** (*MP*) medially and the **masseter** (*MA*) laterally.
- Three superficial back muscles associated with the upper limb appear: **sternocleidomastoid** (*SCM*), **levator scapulae** (*LS*), and **trapezius** (*TZ*).

Clinical Notes

- Tumors of the parotid and other salivary glands may involve the infratemporal region and subsequently invade the parapharyngeal space medial to the pterygoid muscles. This space is the junction of many spaces and a common site for tumor spread.
- Again, the low (dark) MR signal from the cortex of the mandibular ramus (MN2), surrounds the higher (lighter) MR signal from the marrow.

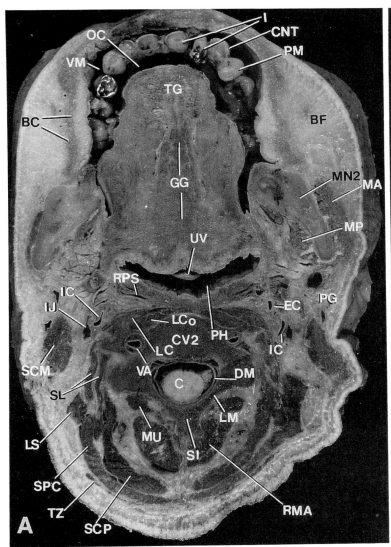

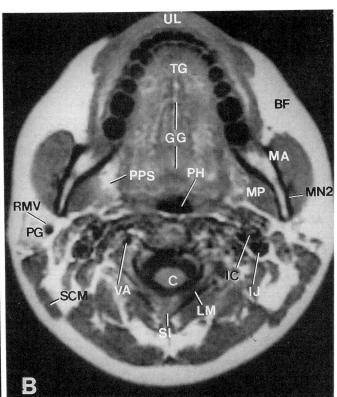

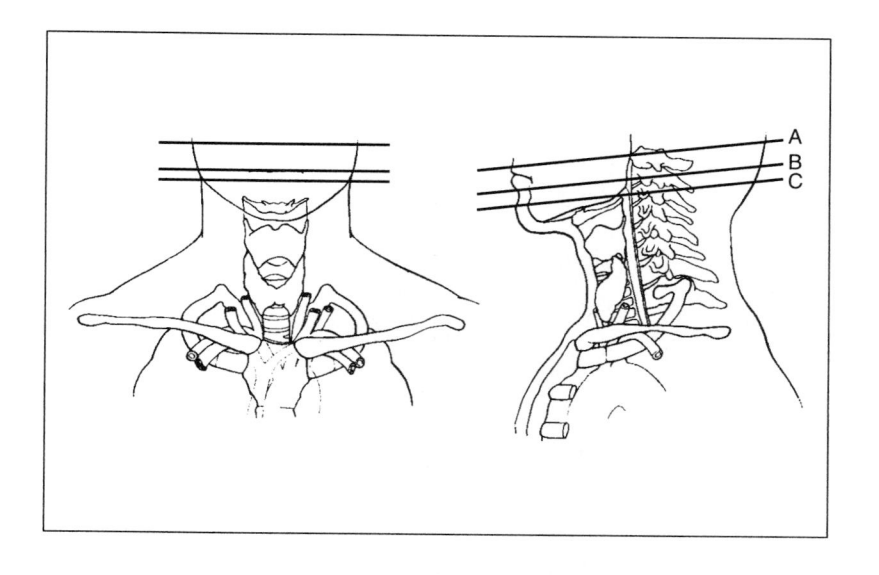

Note

- Sections **A, B,** and **C** in this plate are cut at a slightly oblique angle so that vertebral levels do not correspond exactly with those commonly accepted for placement of the neck organs and vessels.
- The views presented here extend from the **oropharynx** (*PH*) in **A** to the **laryngeal aditus** (*LA*) in **C**.
- The mandible appears first as its **ramus** (*MN2*) in **A** and as the **body** (*MN3*) and **mentis** (*MN4*) in both **B** and **C**. Note how it arches around the floor of the mouth region in the figures presented. In **A**, the **masseter** is lateral to and the **medial pterygoid** (*MP*) medial to the **mandibular ramus** (*MN2*).
- Muscles forming much of the floor of the mouth—**mylohyoid** (*MH*), **geniohyoid** (*GH*) and **hyoglossus** (*HG*)—appear in **B** and **C**. In **C**, the **lingual nerve** (*LNV*) is seen lateral to the **hyoglossus** (*HG*).
- The **submandibular gland** (*SMG*) occupies a position along the posterior edge of the **mylohyoid** (*MH*) and is seen in **B** and **C** and in Plate 24 in **A**. Its confluence with the **parotid gland** (*PG*) is indicated on the right in **B**.
- The **oropharynx** (*PH*) and the region of the **epiglottis** (*EG*), which itself is seen to lie anterior to the **laryngeal aditus** (*AL*) in **C**, appear here.
- Major blood vessels of the head are positionally related to the **cervical vertebrae** (*CV1-CV2*). Coursing along the sides and anterior to the vertebrae are first the **common carotid artery** (*CC*), **B** and **C** and then, in **A**, the terminal branches of this artery, the **external** and **internal carotid arteries** (*EC, IC*).
- The **vertebral artery** (*VA*) lies anterior to the distal part of the **spinal ganglion** (*GN*). This neural structure at the junction of dorsal and ventral nerve roots is in close proximity to the spinal nerve just distal to it, but out of the plane of section here.

Clinical Notes

- The region around the internal jugular vein contains many deep cervical lymph nodes, which often are affected by metastatic head and neck carcinoma. Significant lymphadenopathy may be impalpable, but identification is quite possible with MR imaging or CT scanning.
- MR imaging is useful in detecting lesions within the submandibular gland, tongue, and floor of the mouth and in demonstrating their relationship to the mandible.

References G *7-778, 7-787;* **N** *53, 54, 55;* **RY** *145*

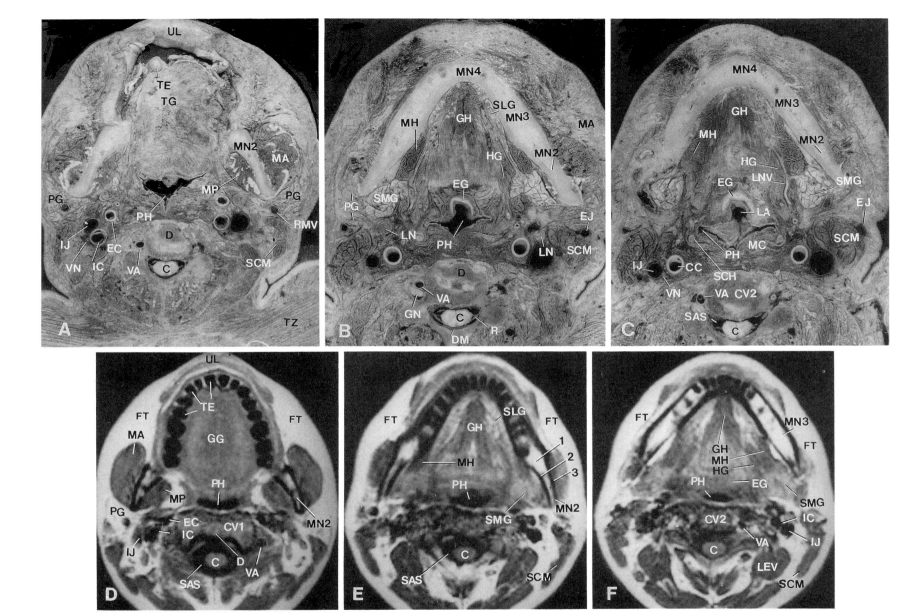

KEY

1 outer table of compact bone of mandible
2 trabecular bone of mandible
3 inner table of compact bone of mandible
C cervical spinal cord
CC common carotid artery

CV1 cervical vertebra 1 (anterior arch)
CV2 cervical vertebra 2
D odontoid process of CV2
DM dura mater
EC external carotid artery
EG epiglottis
EJ external jugular vein
FT buccal fat

GG genioglossus
GH geniohyoid
GN ganglion
HG hyoglossus
IC internal carotid artery
IJ internal jugular vein
LA laryngeal aditus
LEV levator scapulae
LN lymph node

LNV lingual nerve
MA masseter
MC middle pharyngeal constrictor
MH mylohyoid
MN2 ramus of mandible
MN3 body of mandible
MN4 mentis of mandible
MP medial pterygoid

PG parotid gland
PH oropharynx
R dorsal roots of spinal cord
RMV retromandibular vein
SAS subarachnoid space
SCH superior cornu of hyoid bone
SCM sternocleidomastoid
SLG sublingual gland

SMG submandibular gland
TE teeth
TG tongue
TZ trapezius
UL upper lip
VA vertebral artery
VN vagus nerve

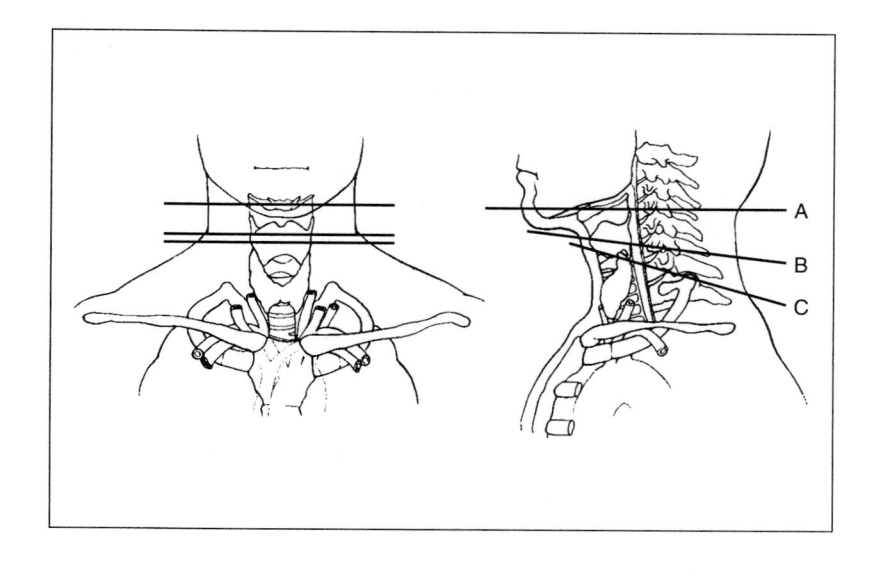

Note

- Sections **A**, **B**, and **C** in this plate are cut at a slightly oblique angle so that vertebral levels do not correspond exactly with those commonly accepted for placement of the neck organs and vessels.
- The sections here extend from the level of the **body of the hyoid bone** (*HY*) to that of the **rima glottidis** (*RG*).
- Parts of the mandibular arch, i.e., **mentis** and **body** (*MN4, MN3*), appear **A**. Also appearing is floor of the mouth musculature continuing from the previous plate and including the **geniohyoid** (*GH*) seen through the cut edges of the **mylohyoid** (*MH*) in **B**. In **A** and **B** the mylohyoid (*MH*) is seen to be flanked bilaterally by the **anterior bellies of the digastric** (*DG*).
- Posterior to the structures already mentioned are the cartilages making up the larynx and including the **lamina of the thyroid cartilage** (*TY*) in **A**, **B**, and **C**, the **cricoid cartilage** (*CRI*) in **C**, and the **arytenoid cartilages** (*ARC*) in **B**. In addition, certain intrinsic muscles of the larynx, including the **posterior cricoarytenoid** (*PC*) in **C**, **transverse arytenoid** (*TA*) in **B**, and the **vocalis** (*VO*) in **C** are seen.
- Just posterolateral to the **thyroid lamina** (*TY*) in **B** and **C** is the upper lobe of the **thyroid gland** (*TYG*).
- Posterior to the laryngeal region lies the **laryngopharynx** (*PH*), whose posterior wall is made up of the **inferior pharyngeal constrictor** (*ICR*).
- Lateral to the laryngeal and pharyngeal regions is a key muscle of the region, the **sternocleidomastoid** (*SCM*), on whose medial side are two major blood vessels of the head and neck, the **common carotid artery** (*CC*) and the **internal jugular vein** (*IJ*). Posteriorly and between these two vessels is the **vagus nerve** (*VN*). Posteromedial to the common carotid artery is the **vertebral artery** (*VA*) in the transverse foramen. These structures are seen in **A**, **B**, and **C**.

Clinical Notes

- The extent of most common laryngeal carcinomas, readily determinable by MR imaging, is critical in choosing between supraglottic laryngectomy, hemilaryngectomy, total laryngectomy, or radiation therapy.
- Coronal MR images through the larynx taken with single breath techniques are extremely useful clinically.

References **G** *8-40, 8-43, 8-45, 8-80;* **N** *72, 73;* **RY** *150, 152, 154, 156, 157, 170, 179.*

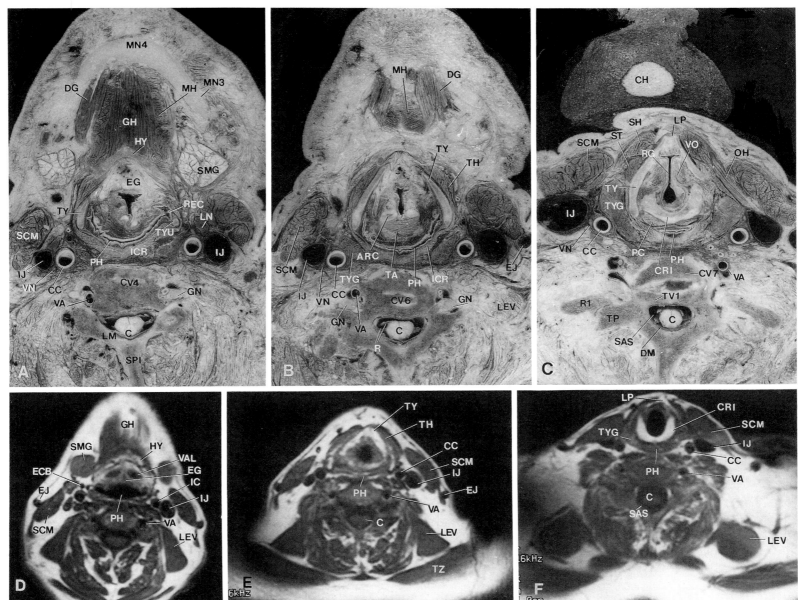

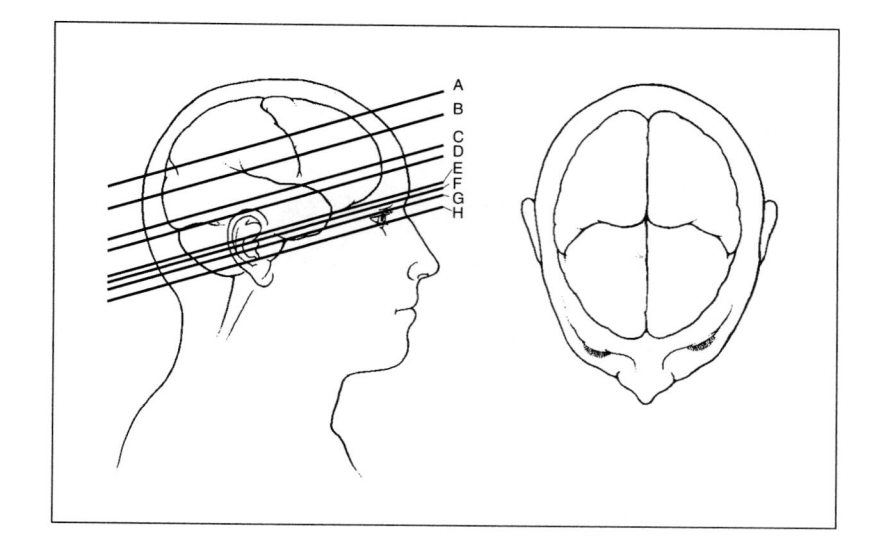

Note

This plate presents T2 and proton density-weighted images which have signals that are different from those seen in T1 images. Notably, the cerebrospinal fluid (CSF) has a high (white) signal. The **caudate nucleus** (*CN*) appears as a gray mass that bulges into the anterior (frontal) horn of the **lateral ventricle** (*LV1*) which, due to its CSF content, appears as a thin white line around the bulge in **C**. Similarly, the **third ventricle** (*TV*) appears as a narrow white line between the **thalami** (*TH*) (left one labeled) in **C** which also shows an expanded part of the subarachnoid space with its CSF, i.e., the **superior vermian cistern** (*SVS*). Vessels, due to flow void signals in both T1 and T2 MR images, appear black. However, other MR sequences can be used to emphasize blood and, depending on the sequence, can make it appear light. The dark signal of the main branch of the **anterior cerebral artery** (*ACA*) is seen in **C**. The **middle cerebral artery** (*MCA*) and the **posterior communicating artery** (*PCA*) are seen in **D**. The course of the **internal carotid artery** (*IC*) can be followed sequentially from its position in the cavernous sinus to its position in the carotid canal in **H**. Numerous smaller **blood vessels** (*BV*), **B,** appear as black wavy lines. White matter is shown to particular advantage as demonstrated by the appearance of the anterior and posterior limbs of the **internal capsule (ICP)** in **C** and the **cerebral peduncles (CPD)** in the mesencephalon (unlabeled) in **D**.

Clinical Note

- T2 images of the cerebrum are anatomically striking and often most sensitive for detection of disease.

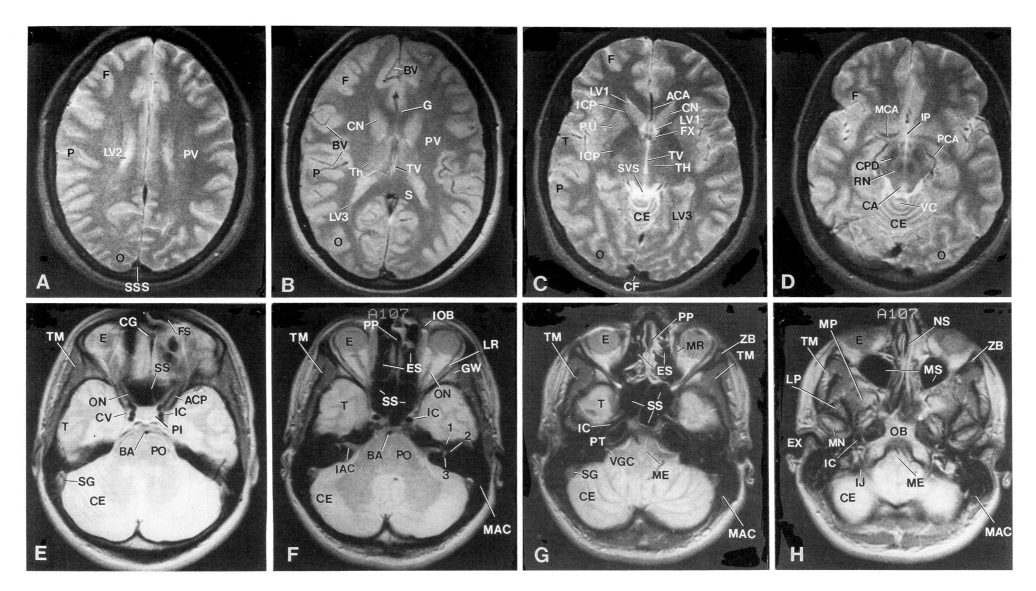

KEY

1 cochlea
2 lateral semicircular canal
3 vestibule
ACA anterior cerebral artery
ACP anterior clinoid process
BA basilar artery
BV blood vessels
CA cerebral aqueduct
CE cerebellum
CF confluence of sinuses
CG crista galli

CN caudate nucleus
CPD cerebral peduncles
CV cavernous sinus
E eyeball
ES ethmoid sinus
EX external auditory meatus
F frontal lobe
FS frontal sinus
FX fornix
G genu of corpus callosum
GW greater wing of sphenoid
IAC internal auditory meatus

IC internal carotid artery
ICP internal capsule
IJ internal jugular
IOB inferior oblique
IP interpeduncular cistern
LP lateral pterygoid
LR lateral rectus
LV1 anterior (frontal) horn, lateral ventricle
LV2 body (parietal horn), lateral ventricle

LV3 posterior (occipital) horn, lateral ventricle
MAC mastoid air cells
MCA middle cerebral artery
ME medulla oblongata
MN head of mandible
MP medial pterygoid
MR medial rectus
MS maxillary sinus
NS nasal septum
O occipital lobe
OB basioccipital bone

ON optic nerve
P parietal lobe
PCA posterior communicating artery
PI pituitary gland
PO pons
PP perpendicular plate
PT petrous temporal bone
PV periventricular white matter
RN red nucleus
S splenium of corpus callosum

SS sphenoid sinus
SSS superior sagittal sinus
SVS superior vermian cistern
T temporal lobe of cerebrum
TH thalamus
TM temporalis muscle
TV third ventricle
VC vermis of cerebellum
VGC confluence of IX,X,XI nerves
ZB zygomatic bone

50

PLATE 26. TV 2-3: clavicle, second part of the subclavian artery, and dome of the pleura: T1 MR image

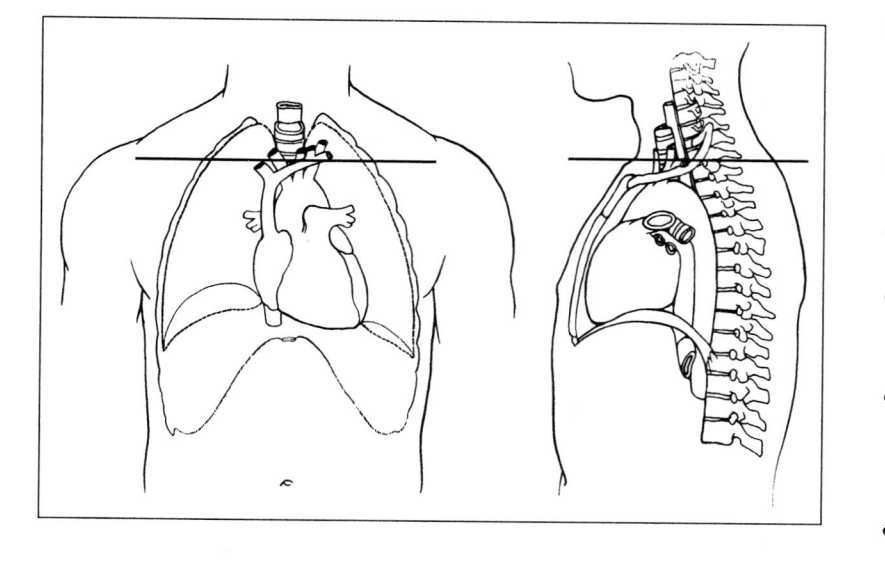

Note

- The surroundings of the junctional region between the root of the neck and the thorax (suprasternal region) include the **clavicle** (CLV), **ribs 1–4** (R1–R4), **second thoracic vertebral body** (TV 2), the **spine of the third thoracic vertebra** (TV 3), and several muscles of the upper limb including the **serratus anterior** (SA), and **pectoralis major** (PM).
- Parts of **Ribs 1–4** (R1–R4) border on the **pleural dome** (PD). The dome is lined by parietal pleura which appears as a transparent, glistening membrane.
- The three major arterial branches of the aortic arch are the **brachiocephalic** (BC), **left common carotid** (CC), and **left subclavian** (SC).
- On the right, the **vagus nerve** (VN) lies between the **brachiocephalic artery** (BC) and the **internal jugular vein** (IJ); on the left (unlabeled), it lies between the left **common carotid artery** (CC) and the **internal jugular vein** (IJ).
- The **anterior scalene** (AS) lies posterior to the **phrenic nerve** (PN), which itself is crossed anteriorly by the **suprascapular artery** (SU). The **second part of the subclavian artery** (SC) lies posterior to the **anterior scalene** (AS) and lateral to it continues as the third part which is enveloped by **portions of the brachial plexus** (BP).
- Close to the midline are the **trachea** (T) and **esophagus** (E) with the **recurrent laryngeal nerve** (RC) running in the groove they form between them.
- The **thoracic spinal cord** (C) is surrounded by the **dura mater** (DM) and **subarachnoid space** (SAS).
- In **B**, which is close to the same plane as **A**, the low signal intensity (black) of the **lungs** (L) is revealed.

Clinical Notes

- The relationship of the superior part of the pleural cavity, the pleural dome, to the clavicle and first rib reveals how penetrating wounds in the root of the neck can injure the lung.
- Trauma or intubation of the trachea may lead to tracheal stenosis, the degree of which is well evaluated by use of MR images in the coronal and sagittal, or often special oblique planes.
- Pancoast (superior sulcus) tumors are bronchogenic carcinomas that arise in the lung apex and often encase adjacent structures.

References **G** *1-15, 1-20, 1-22, 1-23, 1-43, 1-44;* **N** *186, 195, 201, 220;* **RY** *246, 249, 251, 253, 254, 256.*

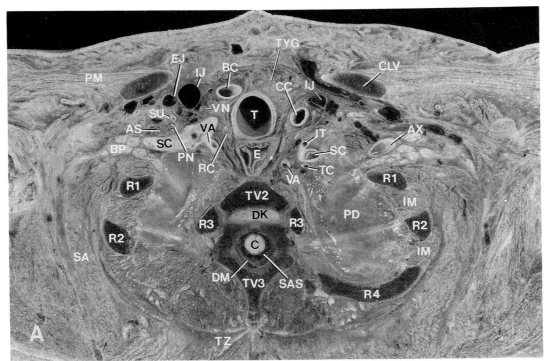

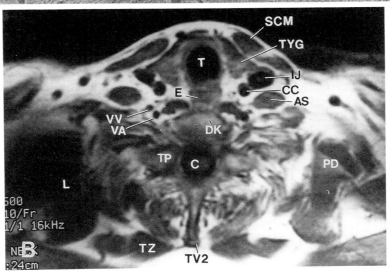

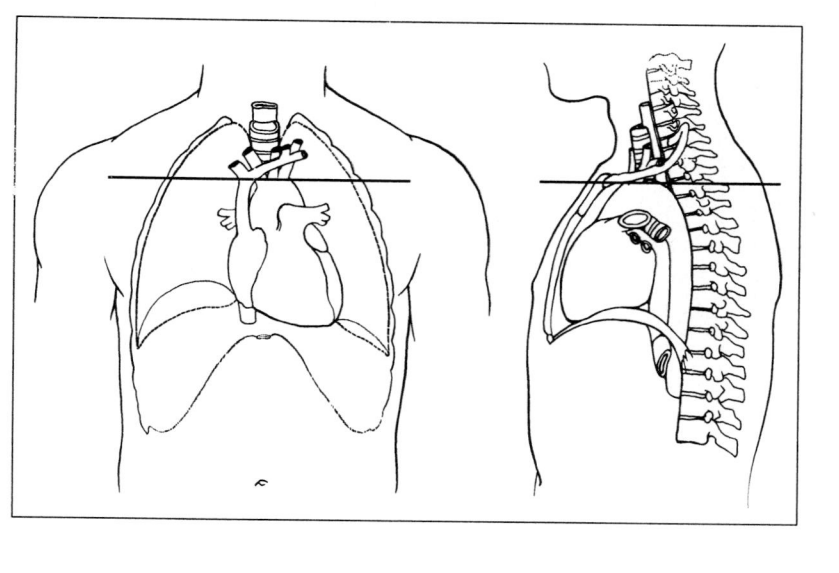

Note

- The surroundings of the thoracic contents at this level include the **manubrium sterni** (*M*), **ribs 2-6** (*R2-6*), **intercostal muscles** (*IM*), **5th thoracic vertebral body** (*TV5*), and muscles of the upper limb including **pectoralis major** (*PM*), **serratus anterior** (*SA*), **latissimus dorsi** (*LD*), **supraspinatus** (*SS*), **infraspinatus** (*IS*), and **trapezius** (*TZ*).
- The **pleural cavity** (*PLC*) lies between the lungs lined by **visceral pleura** (*VP*) and the thoracic wall lined by **parietal pleura** (*PP*).
- The **internal thoracic vessels** (*IT*) are superficial to the **parietal pleura** (*PP*).
- **Pericardial (mediastinal) fat** (*PF*) extends superiorly from the heart region, surrounds the great vessels, and lies between the right and left **pleural cavities** (*PLC*).
- The **brachiocephalic** (*BC*), **left common carotid** (*CC*), and **left subclavian** (*SC*) branches of the **aortic arch** (*AOA*) lie in an anterior to posterior relationship to each other.
- The **superior vena cava** (*SVC*) is anterolateral to the **trachea** (*T*), which itself is anterior to the **esophagus** (*E*).
- In **B**, the **azygos vein** (*AZ*) appears near its termination in the **superior vena cava** (*SVC*).
- **Dura mater** (*DM*) and the **subarachnoid space** (*SAS*) surround the **thoracic spinal cord** (*SC*).

Clinical Notes

- Free-flowing blood generally gives a low-intensity signal (dark) within the vessel, allowing separation of vessels from lymph nodes and other tissue density structures, which have intermediate or higher signal intensity (light).
- MR imaging is generally not used for evaluating lung disease, because signal generation from the relatively minimal amount of tissue present is too low.
- On MR images, cortex of bone has a dark (low) signal, while marrow has a brighter (intermediate) signal (see plates showing cranium). In the case of the scapula which is very thin, the low signals from cortical bone of its internal and external surfaces combine to give a single dark line.

References G *1-76;* **N** *170-230;* **RY** *227-270*

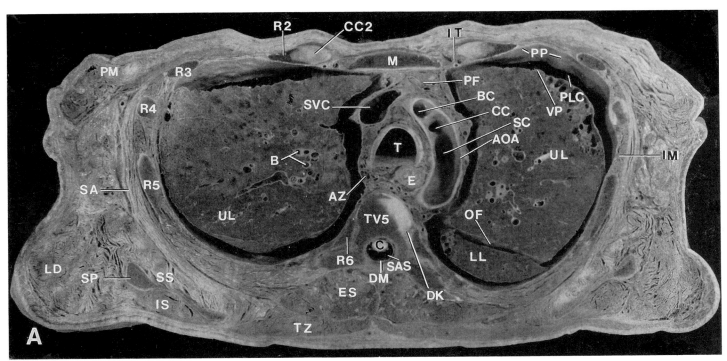

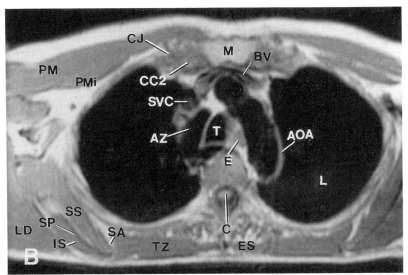

PLATE 28. TV6: junction of superior and middle mediastinum, sternal angle and tracheal bifurcation: T1 MR image

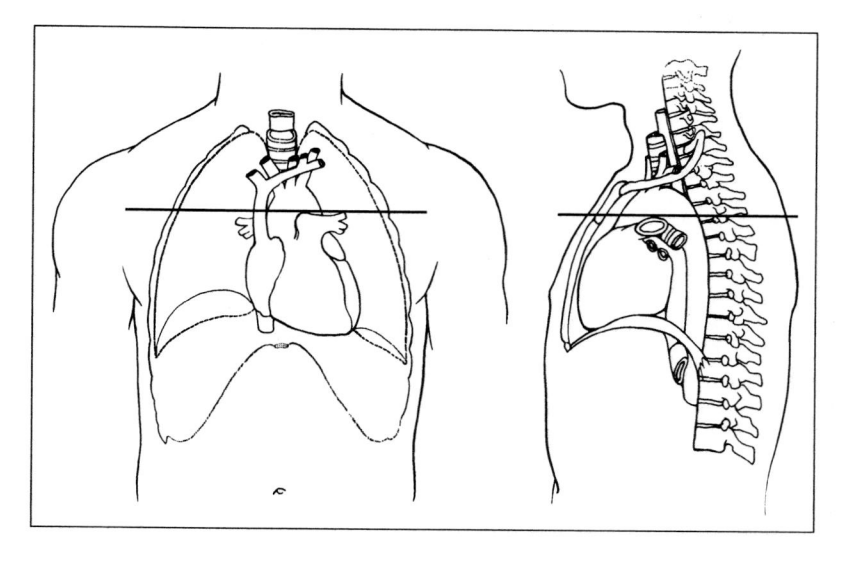

Note

- The surroundings of the thoracic contents at this level include the inferior part of **manubrium sterni** (*M*), **2nd rib costal cartilage** (*CC2*), **third through seventh ribs** (*R3-7*), **intercostal muscles** (*IM*), upper part of the **sixth thoracic vertebral body** (*TV6*), **scapula** (*SP*), and muscles of the upper limb as in the previous plate.
- The **oblique fissures** (*OF*) of both lungs, **visceral** and **parietal** (*VP, PP*) **pleura** and the intervening **pleural cavity** (*PLC*) are seen.
- **Pericardial fat** (*PF*) lined by **parietal pleura** (*PL*) separates left and right **pleural cavities** (*PLC*).
- The **ascending aorta** (*AA*) lies to the left of the **superior vena cava** (*SVC*) and has part of one of the **superior pericardial recesses** (*SR*) to its right.
- The trachea bifurcates into the **right** and **left main bronchi** (*RB*) and (*LB*). The **esophagus** (*E*) lies posterior to the **left main bronchus** (*LB*) and to the right of the **descending aorta** (*DA*); the **azygos vein** (*AZ*) lies posterior to the **right main bronchus** (*RB*).
- A branch of the right **pulmonary artery** (*PA*) lies anterior to the **right main bronchus** (*RB*).

Clinical Notes

- The aortopulmonary window and areas around the tracheal bifurcation are common sites for metastatic adenopathy.
- Breast cancer metastases may be found in lymph nodes adjacent to the internal thoracic blood vessels.
- Thymomas, often occurring in patients with myasthenia gravis, are located in the anterior mediastinum in the area of retrosternal fat. They are often invisible on plain radiographs, but are clearly seen on MR images.

*References **G** 1-76; **N** 170-230; **RY** 227-270*

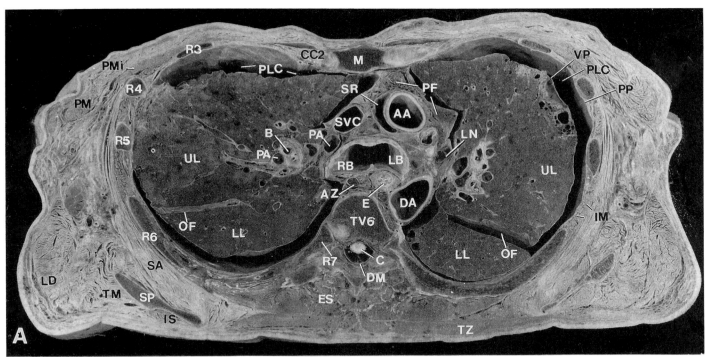

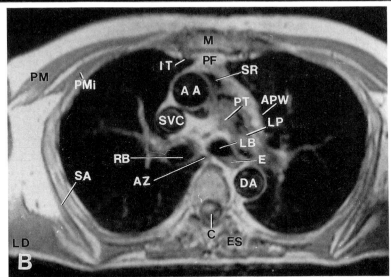

KEY

AA ascending aorta
APW aortopulmonary window
AZ azygos vein
B bronchus
C thoracic spinal cord
CC2 second costal cartilage

DA descending aorta
DM dura mater
E esophagus
ES erector spinae
IM intercostal muscles
IS infraspinatus
IT internal thoracic vessels

LB left main bronchus
LD latissimus dorsi
LL lower lobe of lung
LN lymph node
LP left pulmonary artery
M manubrium sterni
OF oblique fissure

PA pulmonary artery
PF pericardial fat (retrosternal)
PLC pleural cavity
PM pectoralis major
PMi pectoralis minor
PP parietal pleura
PT pulmonary trunk

R3–7 ribs 3–7
RB right main bronchus
SA serratus anterior
SP scapula
SR superior pericardial recess
SVC superior vena cava
TM teres major

TV6 body, thoracic vertebra 6
TZ trapezius
UL upper lobe of lung
VP visceral pleura

PLATE 29. TV7: below aortic arch, ascending and descending aorta, near top of pulmonary artery, inferior angle of scapula: T1 MR image

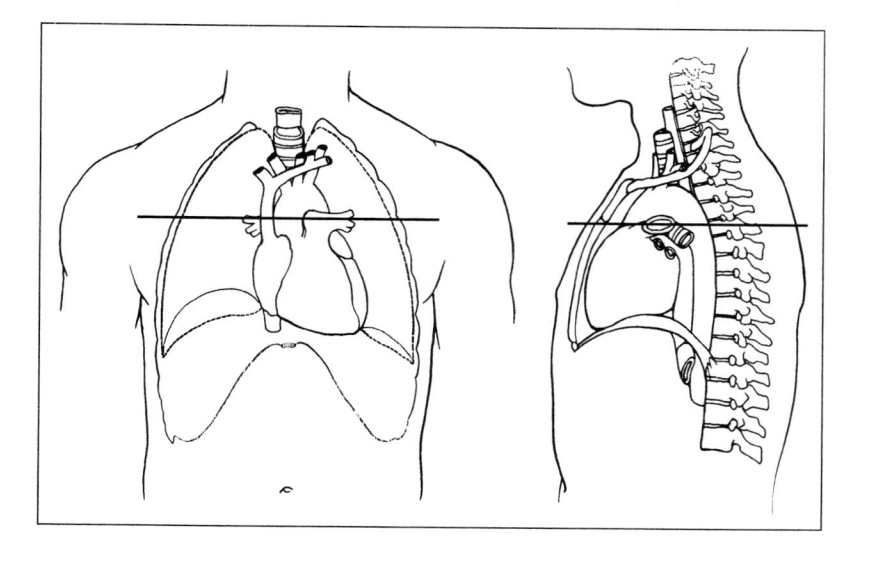

Note

- The surroundings of the thoracic contents at this level include the **sternum** (*ST*), **3rd rib costal cartilage** (*CC3*), **ribs 3–7** (*R3–7*), **intercostal muscles** (*IM*), upper part of the **seventh thoracic vertebral body** (*TV7*), inferior angle of **scapula** (*SP*), and muscles of the upper limb as in the previous plate.
- The lungs, **visceral** and **parietal pleura** (*VP, PP*) and the intervening **pleural cavity** (*PLC*) are seen.
- The **ascending aorta** (*AA*) is surrounded by the **superior pericardial recesses** (*PR*). To its right is the **superior vena cava** (*SVC*). Both vessels are anterior to the **right pulmonary artery** (*RPA*).
- The **right** and the **left main bronchi** (*RB, LB*) are posterior to the **right pulmonary artery** (*RPA*) and between both bronchi, as here, one often finds a **subcarinal lymph node** (*LN*).
- The **azygos vein** (*AZ*) just anterior to the **seventh thoracic vertebral body** (*TV7*), lies to the right of the **esophagus** (*E*), which is anteromedial to the **descending aorta** (*DA*).

Clinical Notes

- It is difficult to visualize the esophagus clearly on imaging studies because often it is collapsed. Occasionally, air in the esophagus allow it to be more clearly visualized as is the case here.
- The four most common anterior mediastinal lesions, which have the appearance of masses or disrupt the portion of the pericardial fat behind the sternum (retrosternal fat), are thymomas, teratomas, substernal thyroids, and lymphomas.
- Compare the signal from blood in the lumen of the pulmonary artery seen in this plate with that of the aorta in the previous plate. Usually the signal from flowing blood is low (dark). The bright signal flow phenomenon in MR images is an effect seen in gating techniques for cardiac MRI.

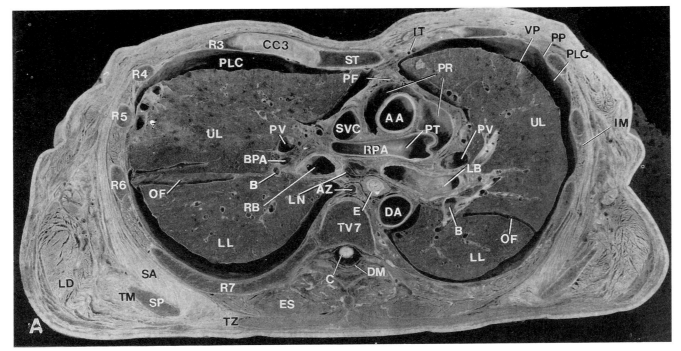

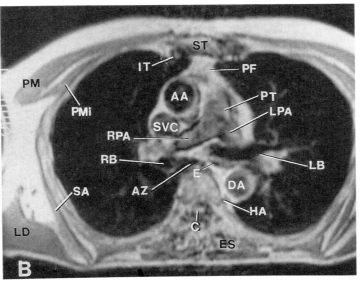

PLATE 30. TV7: sternum, transverse pericardial sinus, pulmonary arteries, and right pulmonary artery: T1 MR image

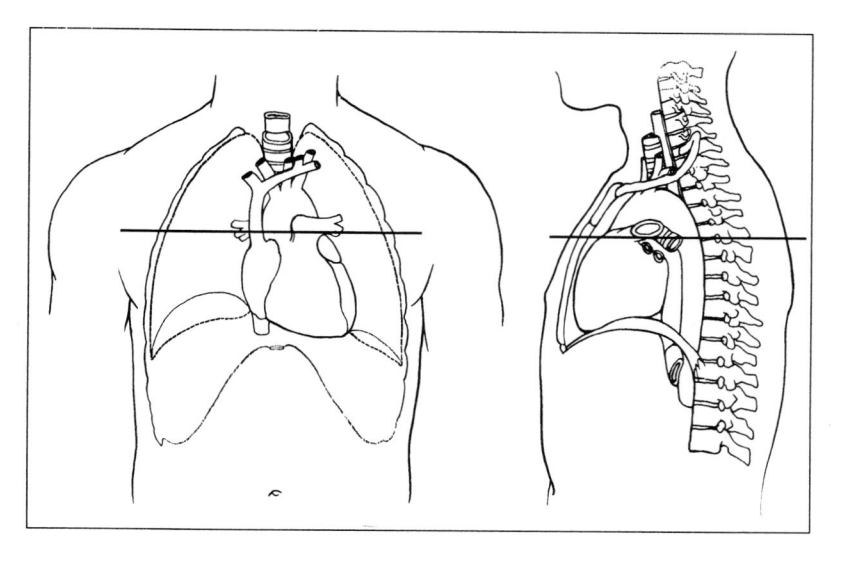

Note

- The surroundings of the thoracic contents at this level include the **sternum** (*ST*), **3rd rib costal cartilage** (*CC3*), **ribs 4–8** (*R4–8*), **intercostal muscles** (*IM*), **TV 7 body** (*TV7*), **inferior angle of scapula** (*SP*), **latissimus dorsi** (*LD*), and **serratus anterior** (*SA*).
- The lungs, **visceral** and **parietal pleura** (*VP, PP*) and the intervening **pleural cavity** (*PLC*) are seen.
- Three structures are aligned from right to left anterior to the **right pulmonary artery** (*RPA*): the **right superior pulmonary vein** (*PV*), **superior vena cava** (*SVC*), and **ascending aorta** (*AA*).
- The lower part of the superior pericardial recess is now more evidently a part of the **pericardial cavity** (*PRC*) and is so named here. The cavity curves from the anteromedial side of the **ascending aorta** (*AA*) around the **pulmonary trunk** (*PT*) to the posterior side of the **right pulmonary artery** (*RPA*) as the **transverse pericardial sinus** (*TPS*).
- The **pericardial fat** (*PF*) lies between the **fibrous (parietal) pericardium** (*FP*) and the **parietal pleura** (*PP*). **Epicardial fat** (*EF*) lies deep to the **epicardium (visceral pericardium)** (*EP*) seen here extending from the region of the heart itself around the lower part of the **ascending aorta** (*AA*) and **pulmonary trunk** (*PT*). See Plate 80 notes, which describe the various linings of the thoracic and abdominal cavities.
- The **azygos vein** (*AZ*) courses here anterior to the **seventh thoracic vertebral body** (*TV7*) and to the right of the **esophagus** (*E*).

Clinical Notes

- Because the left atrial contour occupies the subcarinal region (see Plates 28 and 29) it is sometimes difficult to distinguish left atrial enlargement on CT scans. MR with multiplanar imaging of the flow void phenomenon is ideal to separate flowing blood (**dark signal**) from other tissue densities (**brighter signals**).
- Bronchogenic cysts are often found in the subcarinal area.

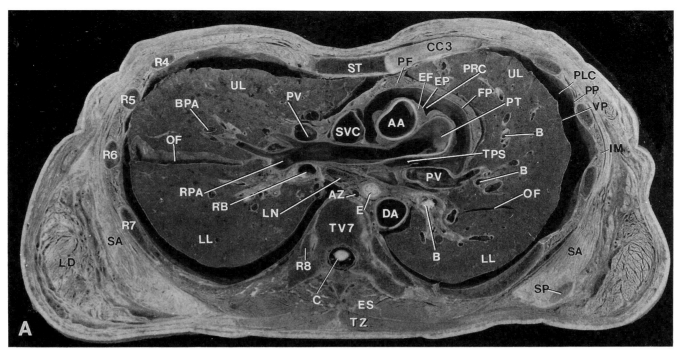

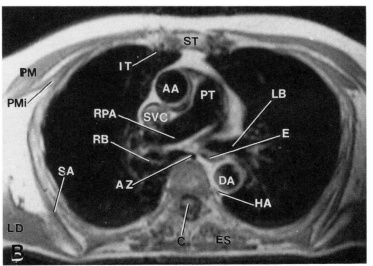

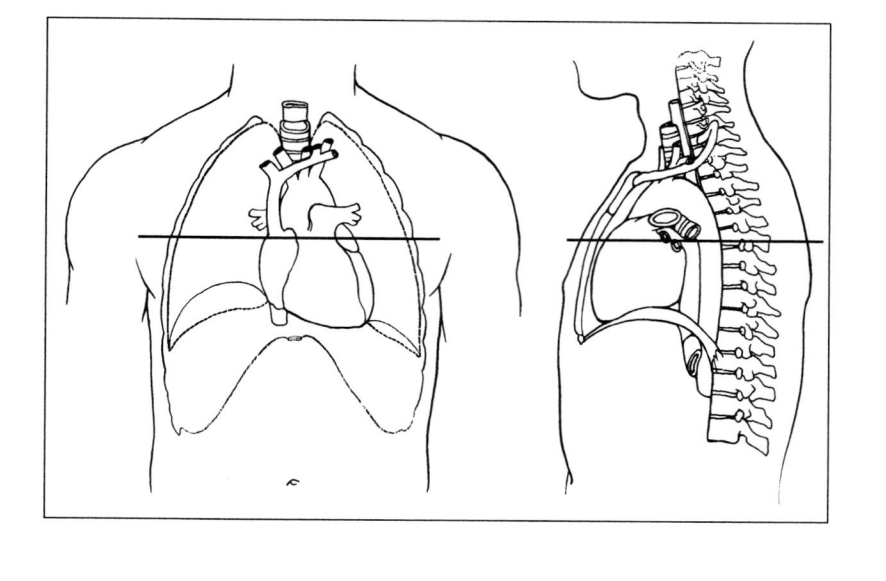

Note

- The surroundings of the thoracic contents at this level include the **sternum** (*ST*), **ribs 4-8** (*R4-R8*), **intercostal muscles** (*IM*), **eighth thoracic vertebral body** (*TV8*), and muscles of the upper limb.
- Four major structures appear in a right to left linear array: **right superior pulmonary vein** (*PV*), **superior vena cava** (*SVC*), **ascending aorta** (*AA*), and **pulmonary trunk** (*PT*).
- The superior portion of the **left atrium** (*LA*) appears posterior to the **ascending aorta** (*AA*), and the **auricle of left atrium** (*LAP*) appears behind the **pulmonary trunk** (*PT*).
- Surrounding the mediastinal structures so far described are the **pericardial fat** (*PF*) associated with the **fibrous pericardium** (*FP*), the **epicardial fat** (*EF*) associated with the epicardium (visceral pericardium) (unlabeled) and the intervening pericardial cavity represented here by two of its subdivisions the **transverse pericardial sinus** (*TPS*) and the superiormost part of the **oblique pericardial sinus** (*OPS*).
- Extending from the left anterolateral edge of the **body of the 8th thoracic veretebra** (*TV8*) and behind the **left atrium** (*LA*) and **oblique pericardial sinus** (*OPS*) are the **azygos vein** (*AZ*), **esophagus** (*E*), and **descending aorta** (*DA*).

Clinical Notes

- The azygos and hemiazygos veins are seen approximately 90% of the time in MR images. Any other structures, usually of intermediate density, especially those greater than 7-10 mm in diameter, are considered to be abnormal lymph nodes.

References **G** *1-76;* **N** *170-230;* **RY** *227-270*

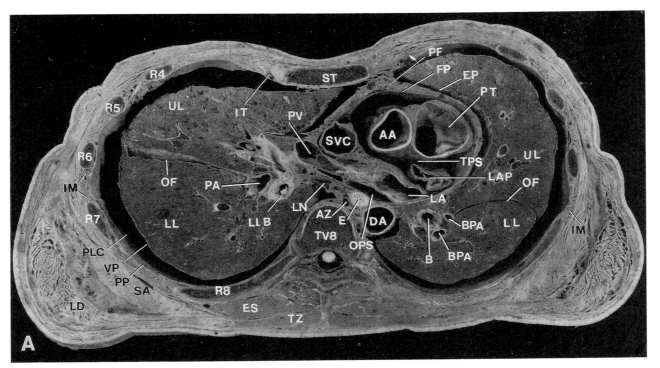

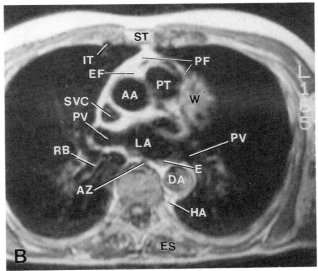

PLATE 32. TV8: sternum, oblique pericardial sinus, pulmonary valve: T1 MR image

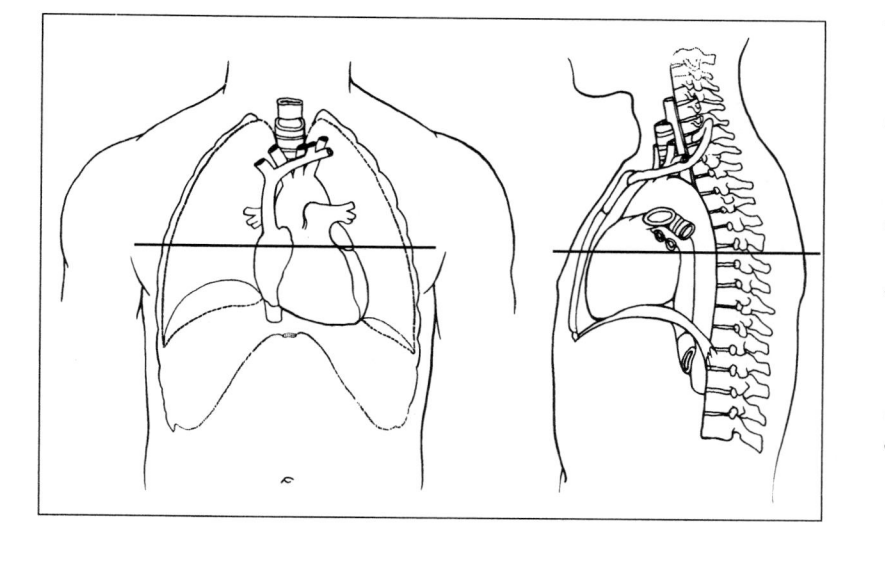

Note

- The surroundings of the thoracic contents at this level include the **sternum** (*ST*), **ribs 5-8** (*R5-R8*), **intercostal muscles** (*IM*), **8th thoracic vertebral body** (*TV8*), and muscles of the upper limb, including the **latissimus dorsi** (*LD*) and **serratus anterior** (*SA*).
- Structures at the base of the heart include centrally the aortic orifice marked by the **aortic valve** (*AV*). To its left is the **pulmonary valve** (*PVA*), to its right the **superior vena cava** (*SVC*), posteriorly, the **left atrium** (*LA*), and anteriorly, the **auricle of right atrium** (*RAP*).
- The **right pulmonary vein** (*RPV*), which is posterior to the **superior vena cava** (*SVC*), opens into the **left atrium** (*LA*).
- Extending from the left anterolateral edge of the **body of the 8th thoracic vertebra** (*TV8*) and behind the **left atrium** (*LA*) and **oblique pericardial sinus** (*OPS*) the **azygos vein** (*AZ*), **esophagus** (*E*), and **descending aorta** (*DA*) are seen.

Clinical Notes

- Pericardial fat is coextensive with the fibrous pericardium, which extends superiorly and covers the beginnings of the great vessels and appears in this MR image. Note that pericardial fat is anatomically and clinically differentiated from the epicardial fat, which lies deep to the mesothelium of the visceral pericardium. The pericardial cavity, clinically most often a potential space, when enlarged (as is not the case in this MRI) appears black and is well seen when contrasted between the pericardial and epicardial fat.

References G 1-76; N 170-230; RY 227-270

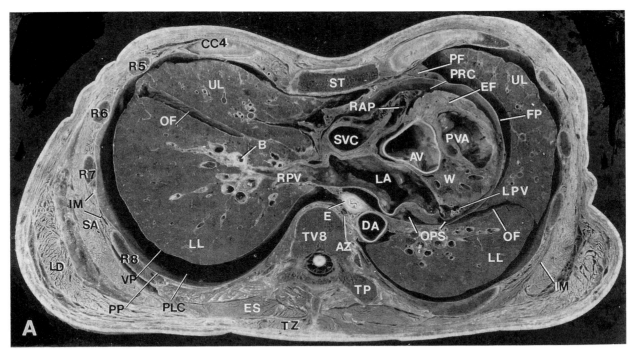

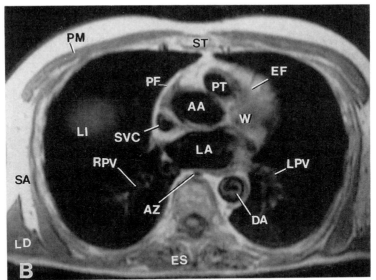

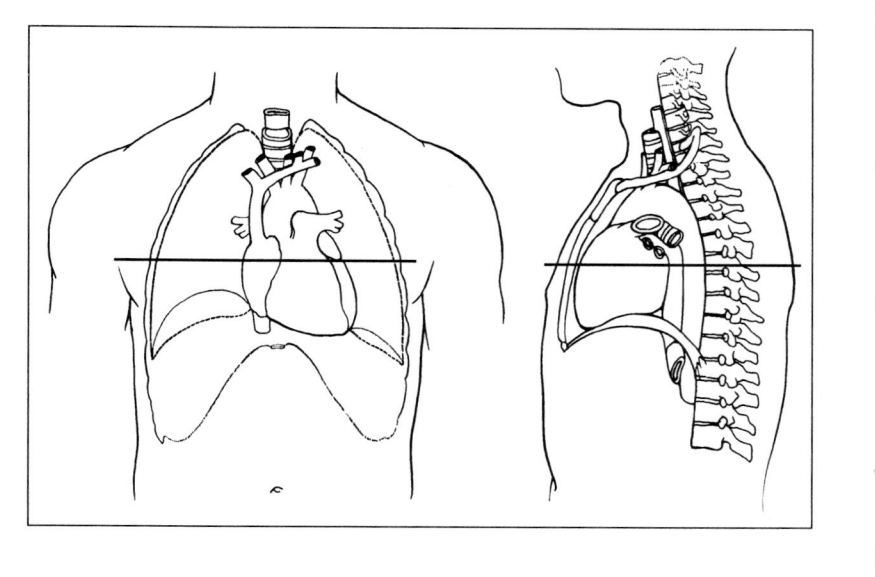

Note

- The surroundings of the thoracic contents at this level include the **sternum** (*ST*), **costal cartilages of ribs 6-7** (*CC6-CC7*), **ribs 4-9** (*R4-R9*), **intercostal muscles** (*IM*), **9th thoracic veretebra** (*TV9*), and muscles of the upper limb, including **latissimus dorsi** (*LD*), **serratus anterior** (*SA*), and **pectoralis major** (*PM*).

- All of the heart chambers appear here. Located centrally is the upper part of the **left ventricle** (*LV*) at the **aortic valve** (*AV*) as well as the **tricuspid valve** (*TV*). Posterior to the **left ventricle** (*LV*) is the **left atrium** (*LA*); anterior to it is the **right ventricle** (*RV*); to its right is the **right atrium** (*RA*). The right atrium here is very close to the entrance of the superior vena cava.

- All the serous linings and spaces of the thoracic cavity appear here. Associated with the lungs are the **parietal** and **visceral pleurae** (*PP, VP*) and the intervening **pleural cavity** (*PLC*); associated with the heart and its great vessels, are the **visceral pericardium (epicardium)** (*EP*), **pericardial cavity** (*PRC*), **parietal pericardium (fibrous pericardium)** (*FP*), and the endocardially lined heart chambers, i.e., **left atrium** (*LA*), **left ventricle** (*LV*), **right ventricle** (*RV*), and **right atrium** (*RA*).

- Muscles of the anterior abdominal wall make their appearance at this level and include the **rectus abdominis** (*RAB*) and the **external abdominal oblique** (*EO*).

Clinical Notes

- Both the thin right atrial wall and the right ventricular wall contrast sharply with that of the left ventricle. Dynamic MR imaging (i.e., images obtained during specific phases of the cardiac cycle) is currently being investigated for the evaluation of cardiac function.

- This plate illustrates one of the difficulties of attempting to match cadaver sections with patient MR images. Here, note that the liver makes its appearance in the MR images at a level somewhat higher than in the cadaver. This results because the liver in cadavers assumes a lower position. Note also that the heart in the cadaver sections is somewhat enlarged, while that of the patient in the MR image is of normal size.

References G *1-76;* **N** *170-230;* **RY** *227-270*

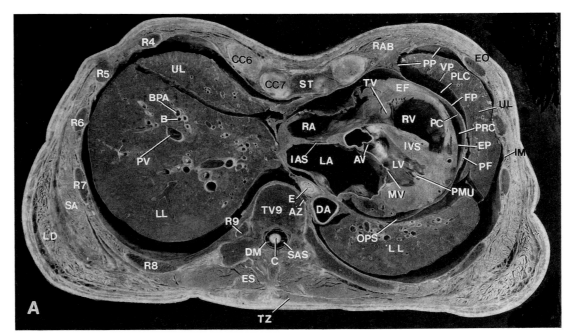

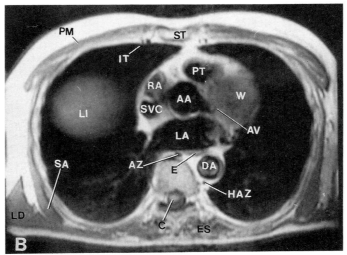

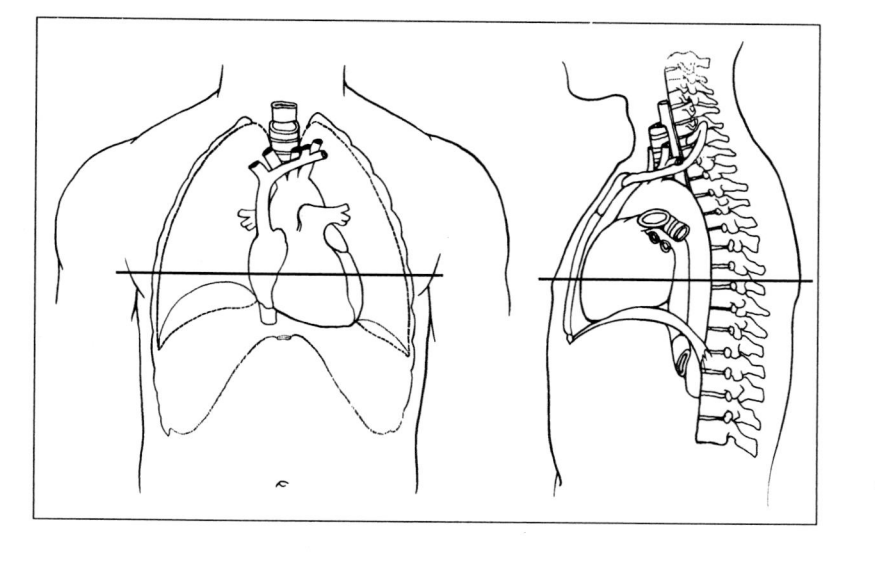

Note

- The surroundings of the thoracic contents at this level include the **subcostal angle** (*white dots*), **costal cartilages of ribs 5-7** (*CC5-CC7*), **ribs 5-9** (*R5-R9*), **intercostal muscles** (*IM*), **intervertebral disk between the 9th and 10th thoracic vertebra** (*TV9*), muscles of the upper limb, **latissimus dorsi** (*LD*) and **serratus anterior** (*SA*), and muscles of the anterior abdominal wall, **rectus abdominis** (*RAB*) and **external abdominal oblique** (*EO*).
- The lungs, **visceral** and **parietal pleura** (*VP, PP*) and the intervening **pleural cavity** (*PLC*) are seen.
- The chambers of the heart are all seen here. Posteriorly are the **left ventricle** (*LV*) and **left atrium** (*LA*), separated by the **mitral valve** (*MV*). Anteriorly are the **right ventricle** (*RV*) and the **right atrium** (*RA*), separated by the **tricuspid valve** (*TV*).
- The **coronary sinus** (*CS*) lies between the **descending aorta** (*DA*) and the **left atrium** (*LA*).
- The **azygos vein** (*AZ*), esophagus (*E*), and **descending aorta** (*DA*) are found posterior to the **oblique pericardial sinus** (*OPS*) and **left atrium** (*LA*).

Clinical Notes

- In various types of heart disease, an enlarged left atrium may press posteriorly into the posterior mediastinum. This is seen as an esophageal constriction or extrinsic indentation on the barium swallow x-ray examination, and is also visible in MR images and CT scans.

References G 1-76; N 170-230; RY 227-270

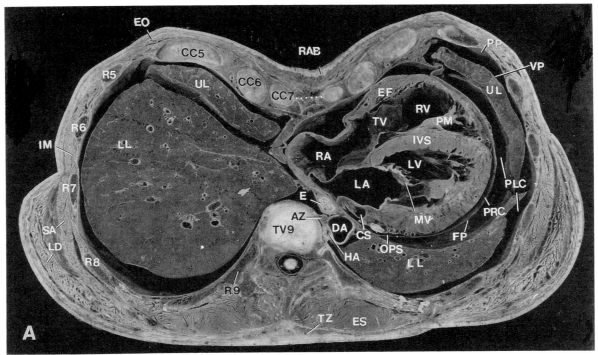

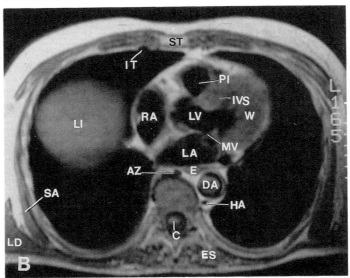

AZ azygos vein
C thoracic spinal cord
CC5–7 costal cartilages of ribs 5–7
CS coronary sinus
DA descending aorta
E esophagus

EF epicardial fat
EO external abdominal oblique
ES erector spinae
FP fibrous pericardium
HA hemiazygos vein
IM intercostal muscles

IT internal thoracic vessels
IVS interventricular septum
LA left atrium
LD latissimus dorsi
LI liver
LL lower lobe of lung
LV left ventricle

MV mitral valve
OPS oblique pericardial sinus
PI pulmonary infundibulum
PLC pleural cavity
PM papillary muscle
PP parietal pleura
PRC pericardial cavity

R5–9 ribs 5–9
RA right atrium
RAB rectus abdominis
RV right ventricle
SA serratus anterior
ST sternum
TV tricuspid valve

TV9 disk between thoracic vertebrae 9 and 10
TZ trapezius
UL upper lobe of lung
VP visceral pleura
W left ventricular wall
White dots subcostal angle

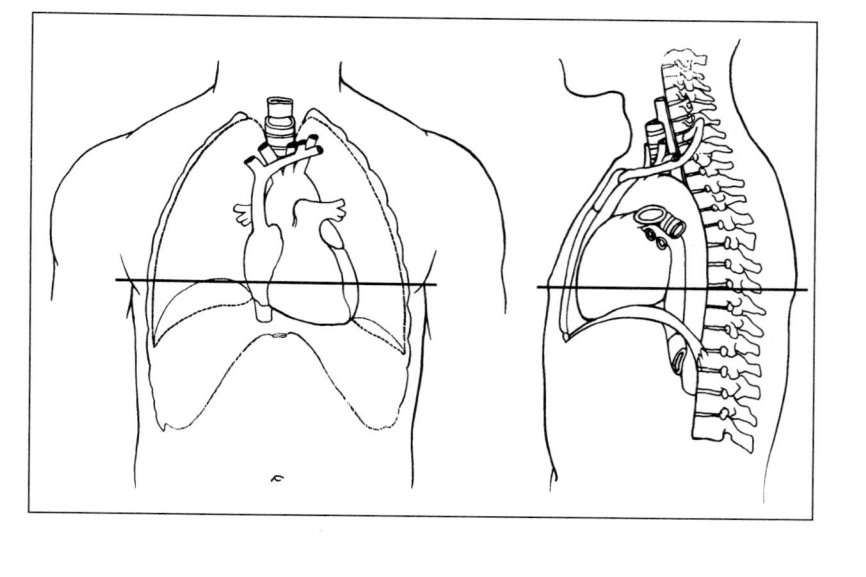

Note

- The surroundings of the thoracic contents at this level include the **subcostal angle** (*white dots*), **costal cartilages of ribs 6 and 7** (*CC6-CC7*), **ribs 6-10** (*R6-R10*), **intercostal muscles** (*IM*), **TV10 body** (*TV10*), muscles of the upper limb, **latissimus dorsi** (*LD*) and **serratus anterior** (*SA*), and muscles of the anterior abdominal wall, **rectus abdominis** (*RAB*) and **external abdominal oblique** (*EO*).
- Three of the four chambers of the heart are seen: **left ventricle** (*LV*), near the apex of the heart, **right ventricle** (*RV*) and **right atrium** (*RA*) at the entrance of the **inferior vena cava** (*IVC*), which is marked by the presence of the **valve of the inferior vena cava** (*V*).
- The **descending aorta** (*DA*) and **esophagus** (*E*), which more superiorly were posterior to the left atrium, are here posterior to the **right atrium** (*RA*).
- Observation of the epicardial fat reveals the location of coronary arteries. Anteriorly, designated by *CA1*, is a branch of the **right coronary artery**. Laterally, at the inferior extent of the interventricular septum at *CA2* is a branch of the **left anterior descending coronary artery**.

Clinical Notes

- The coronary arteries lie in the epicardial fat and are often well visualized in MR images.

*References G 1-76; **N** 170-230; **RY** 227-270*

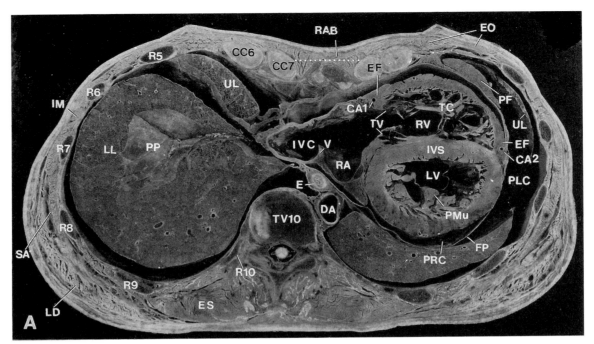

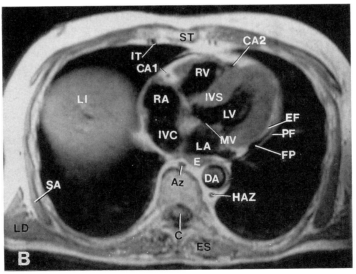

PLATE 36. TV10-TV11: costodiaphragmatic region, pleural, pericardial, and peritoneal cavities, right lobe of the liver: T1 MR image

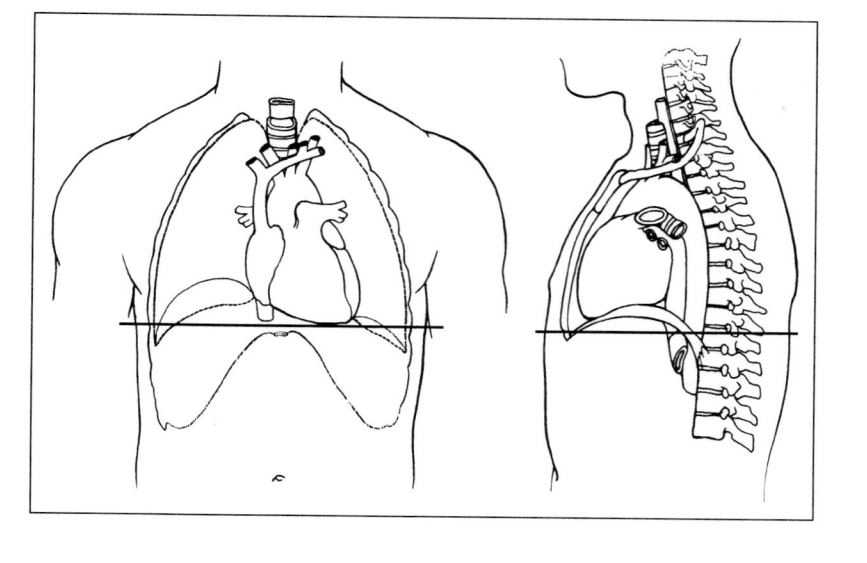

Note

- The surroundings of the thoracic contents at this level include the space marking the **subcostal angle** (*white dots*), **fifth costal cartilages** (*CC5*), **ribs 6-10** (*R6-R10*), **intercostal muscles** (*IM*), **disk between the 10th and 11th thoracic vertebra** (*TV10*), anterolateral abdominal musculature including the **rectus abdominis** (*RAB*) and **external abdominal oblique** (*EO*).
- The **pericardial** (*PRC*), **pleural** (*PLC*), and **peritoneal** (*PEC*) cavities with their related coverings are seen here. The pleural cavity is lined by parietal pleura and the lungs by visceral pleura. The external part of the heart is lined by epicardium (visceral pericardium), which reflects on to fibrous pericardium (parietal pericardium), forming a sac around the heart. Between the epicardium and the fibrous pericardium is the pericardial cavity. Similarly, the liver, here, the **right lobe of the liver** (*RL*) lies in the upper part of the **peritoneal cavity** (*PEC*). The liver is lined by visceral peritoneum except on its bare area, and the **diaphragm** (*DI*) is lined by parietal peritoneum on much of its abdominal surface. On its thoracic cavity surface, it is lined by parietal pleura. In this region, the **pleural cavity** (*PLC*) is narrow where it forms the anterior and posterior **costophrenic recesses** (*CPR*).
- The region near the **apex of the heart** (*AX*) is seen through the cut edges of the **fibrous pericardium** (*FP*). It is covered by a glistening layer of epicardium (visceral pericardium, not labeled).
- The **right and left hepatic veins** (*RH, LH*) enter the **inferior vena cava** (*IVC*).
- The **cardiac portion of the stomach** (*CS*) lies just anterior to the **abdominal aorta** (*AB*), which itself is just lateral to the **azygos vein** (*AZ*).
- The upper part of the **right lobe of the liver** (*RL*) lies adjacent to the cut edges of the **diaphragm** (*DI*).

Clinical Notes

- In various lung diseases, pleural fluid often fills the costophrenic spaces and is removed by thoracentesis (percutaneous needle aspiration). The proximity of the lung and the liver on the right, and the lung and spleen on the left shows how the liver, an abdominal organ, may easily be injured in attempts to remove fluid from the pleural cavity or in thoracic wall trauma.
- The normally thin diaphragm is poorly visualized by sectional imaging techniques such as MR and CT.
- Visualization of the flow void within the hepatic veins and hepatic vein confluence is crucial in excluding hepatic vein thrombosis (Budd-Chiari syndrome).
- The pleural fat, when more extensive, can mimic a pleural-based lesion such as asbestosis on plain radiographs.

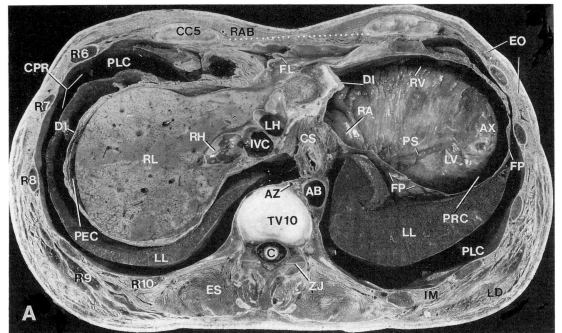

A

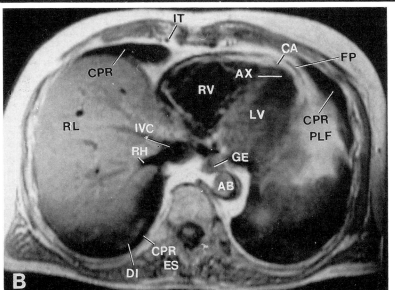

B

KEY

AB abdominal aorta
AX apex of heart
AZ azygos vein
C thoracic spinal cord
CA coronary artery
CC5 fifth costal cartilage

CPR costophrenic recess
CS cardiac stomach
DI diaphragm
EO external abdominal oblique
ES erector spinae
FL falciform ligament

FP fibrous pericardium
GE gastroesophageal junction
IM intercostal muscles
IT internal thoracic vessels
IVC inferior vena cava
LD latissimus dorsi
LH left hepatic vein

LL lower lobe of lung
LR right lobe of liver
LV left ventricle (wall)
PEC peritoneal cavity
PLC pleural cavity
PLF pleural fat
PRC pericardial cavity

PS posterior interventricular sulcus
R6–10 ribs 6–10
RA right atrium (wall)
RAB rectus abdominis
RH right hepatic vein
RL right lobe of liver

RV right ventricle (wall)
TV10 body, thoracic vertebra 10
ZJ facet joint (zygoapophyseal joint)
White dots subcostal angle

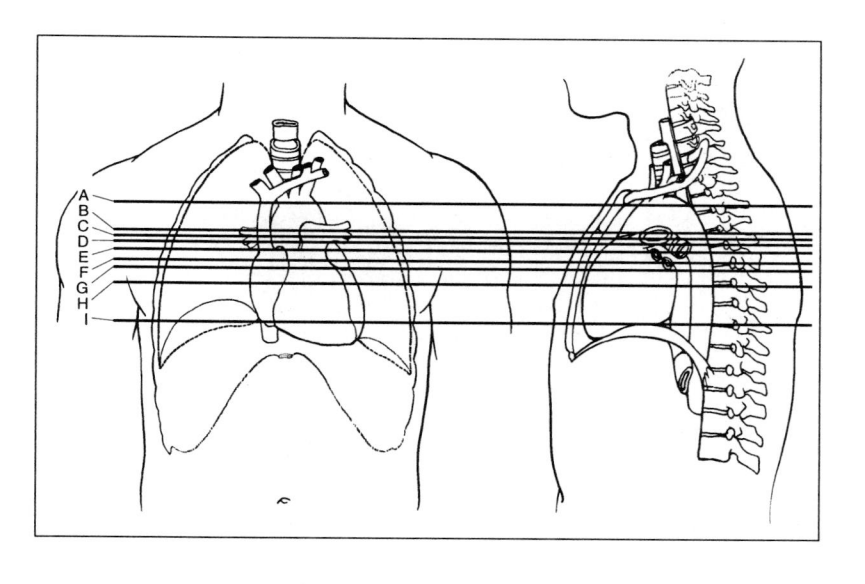

Note

A review of the plate below emphasizes the usefulness of sequential image plates in following the course of certain structures. The images here fall into three regions: superior mediastinum **A-C**, the junction of the superior and inferior mediastinum (sternal angle, **D**), and the inferior mediastinum (anterior, middle, and posterior mediastinum, **E-I**). Concentrating on the course of the aorta allows one to conceptually understand the relationships of parts. It is first observed at its **arch** (*AOA*) and subsequently in its **ascending** (*AA*) and **descending** (*DA*) portions **B-H**. In **G**, the **ascending aorta** (*AA*) disappears as it arises from the **left ventricle** (*LV*), but the **descending aorta** (*DA*) continues through **I** close to where it passes through the diaphragm to become the abdominal aorta (see previous plate). Important relationships inferior to the arch and/or between the ascending and descending portions of the aorta are as follows. In **A** and **B**, the most posterior structures are the **trachea** (*T*) or its **bifurcation** (*RB, LB* in *B*), and the **esophagus** (*E*). In **E-I**, below the sternal angle, the **left atrium** (*LA*) lies posteriorly, with the **esophagus** (*E*) behind it. Close to the diaphragm, as the **left atrium** (*LA*) ends, the **right atrium** (*RA*) assumes its position anterior to the **esophagus** (*E*). The **azygos vein** (*AZ*) lies just to the right of the **esophagus** (*E*) for most of its course before it passes further to the right and anteriorly to enter the **superior vena cava** (*SVC*) in **A**.

Clinical Notes

Observing multiple images allows one to define the location and extent of structures more accurately or the degree to which pathological processes have involved a region. Sequential images of the thorax are particularly necessary in the clinical setting because of the frequency of occurrence of anatomical variations in the course of longitudinally oriented structures.

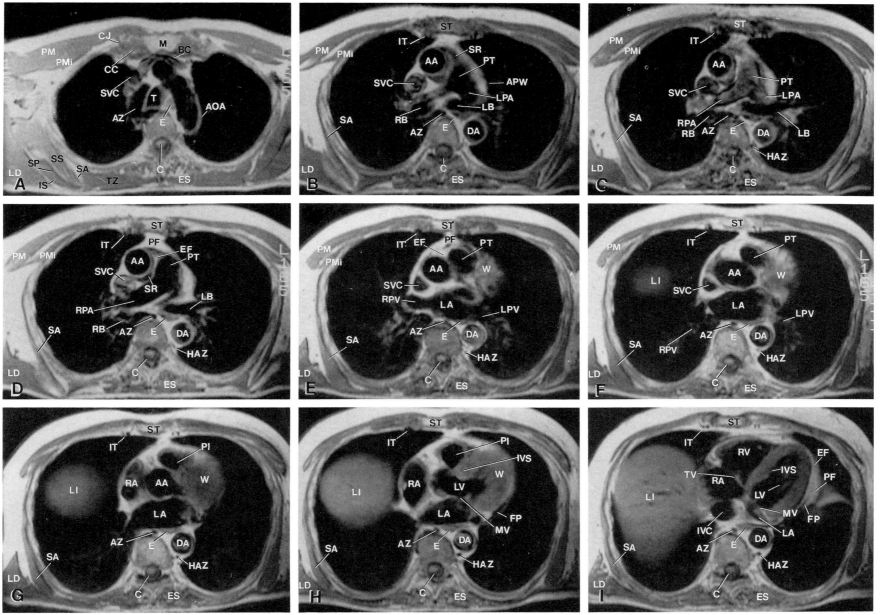

PLATE 38. TV12: lower part of costodiaphragmatic recesses, liver at porta hepatis, and spleen: CT scan, oral iodinated contrast

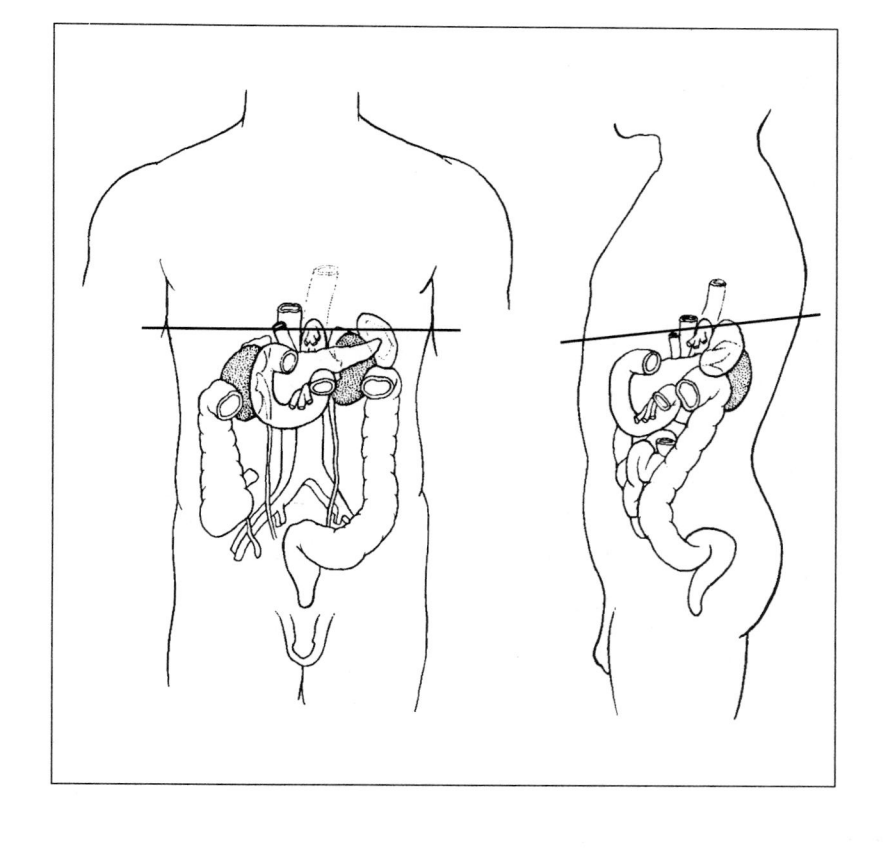

Note

- **B** is from a less muscular patient and is inferior to **A,** which is cut slightly obliquely, thus passing superior to the kidneys.
- The surroundings of the abdominal contents at this level include the **12th thoracic vertebra** (*TV12*), the **erector spinae** (*ES*), **ribs 8-10** (*R8-R10*), **intercostal muscles** (*IM*), muscles of the upper limb, **serratus anterior** (*SA*) and **latissimus dorsi** (*LD*), and anterolateral abdominal muscles, **external abdominal oblique** (*EO*) and **transversus abdominis** (*TA*).
- Along the sides of the vertebral body are the posterior abdominal muscles, **psoas major** (*PM*) and **quadratus lumborum** (*QL*).
- The **peritoneal cavity** (*PEC*) lies between the **visceral peritoneum** (*VP*) and the **parietal peritoneum** (*PAP*), covering the inside walls of the abdominal cavity. The peritoneal cavity is normally a narrow space that is not well seen by imaging techniques. Here, in the wet specimen, its seemingly wide appearance is due to artifactual shrinkage of the abdominal organs after death.
- The **right** and **left lobes of the liver** (*RL, LL*) are seen in their relationship to the **portal vein** (*PV*), which itself lies anterior to the **inferior vena cava** (*IVC*).
- The right **adrenal gland** (*AG*) lies posterolateral to the **inferior vena cava** (*IVC*) in **A**. The left **adrenal gland** (*AG*) lies between the **body of the stomach** (*BS*) and the **abdominal aorta** (*AB*) in **A** and **B**.
- The **body of the stomach** (*BS*) lies posterior to the **left lobe of the liver** (*LL*) and anterior to the **spleen** (*SP*).
- The **celiac artery** (*CA*) is the first midline abdominal branch of the **abdominal aorta** (*AB*).
- Through the cut edges of the **diaphragm** (*DI*), the **right posterior costophrenic recess** (*CPR*) is seen.
- The **sacral spinal cord** (*C*), sectioned near the conus medullaris, is surrounded by portions of the **cauda equina** (*EQ*), occupying the cranial limit of the lumbar cistern. The **dura mater** (*DM*) forms the sac that surrounds this expanded portion of the **subarachnoid space** (*SAS*). The arachnoid membrane is too thin to be visualized even in the wet specimen.

Clinical Notes

- Fat planes surrounding the celiac and superior mesenteric arteries are preferential sites for the spread of pancreatic cancer.
- The adrenal glands are often the site of metastasis from lung cancer. This can be shown on T1 MR images and is usually an inoperable condition.
- The oblique fissure of the liver is often, but not always, the location of the gallbladder (see Plate 40).

References G 78-146; N 231-333; RY 271-302

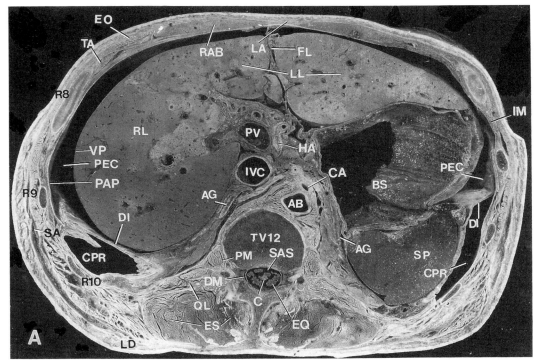

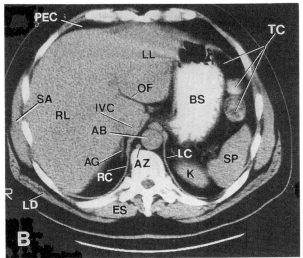

PLATE 39. LV1: left and right lobes of liver, spleen, and head of pancreas: CT scan, oral iodinated contrast

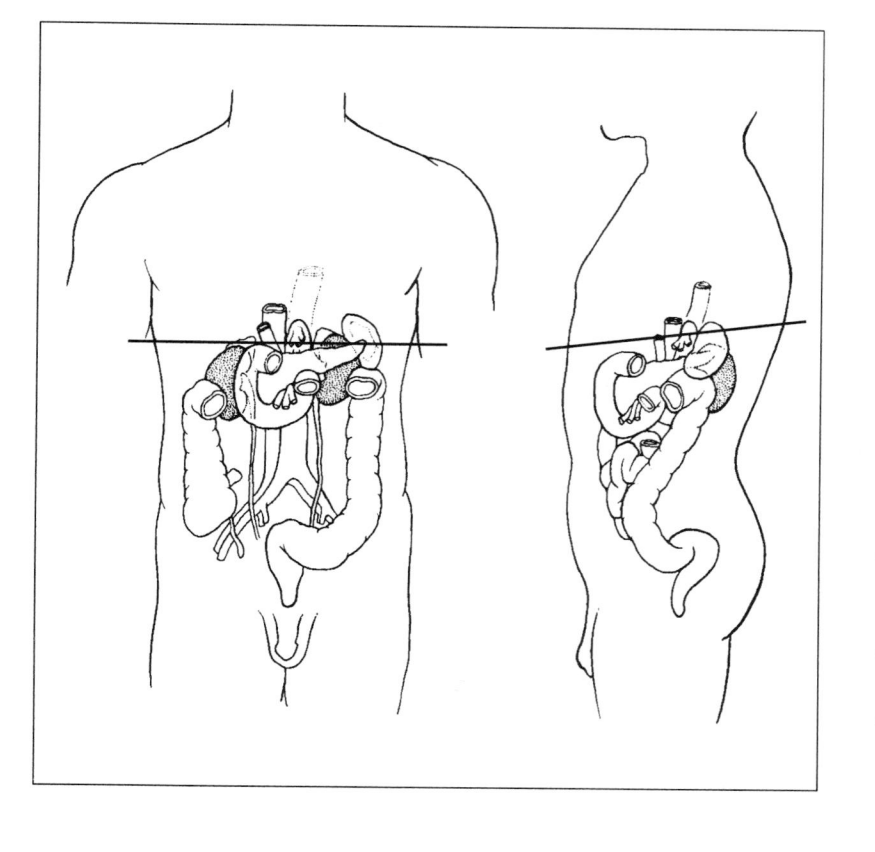

Note

- The surroundings of the abdominal contents at this level include the **first lumbar vertebra** (*LV1*), **erector spinae** (*ES*), **psoas major** (*PM*), and **quadratus lumborum** (*QL*), **ribs 9-10** (*R9-R10*), **intercostal muscles** (*IM*), anterolateral abdominal muscles, **rectus abdominis** (*RAB*), **external abdominal oblique** (*EO*), **internal abdominal oblique** (*IO*), and **transversus abdominis** (*TA*).
- The **right and left lobes of the liver** (*RL, LL*), separated by the **oblique fissure** (*OF*), lie on either side of the **first and second parts of the duodenum** (*D1, D2*), just as the second part begins its descent along the lateral border of the **head of the pancreas** (*P1*).
- The **portal vein** (*PV*), adjacent to the **head of the pancreas** (*P1*), is anterior to the **inferior vena cava** (*IVC*).
- The **spleen** (*SP*) is posterior to the **body of the stomach** (*BS*), which itself is posterior to the **left lobe of the liver** (*LL*).
- The **left adrenal gland** (*AG*) is embedded in **perirenal fat** (*PF*) and lies between the **splenic vein** (*SV*) and **abdominal aorta** (*AB*). The **right adrenal gland** (*AG*) is almost out of the plane of section and lies posterior to the **inferior vena cava** (*IVC*).

Clinical Notes

- Without using intravenous contrast, it is often impossible on CT scans to differentiate the portal vein from the head of the pancreas, or to distinguish lymph nodes from blood vessels or other tissue (see also IVC adjacent to liver in Plate 38B).
- The falciform ligament separates the medial from the lateral segment of the left lobe of the liver (*double arrow* in **B**).
- In CT scans, fat has a low density and appears black, as seen here in the perirenal fat.

References **G** *78-146;* **N** *231-333;* **RY** *271-302*

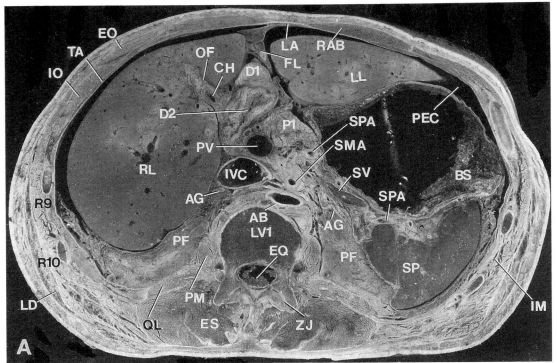

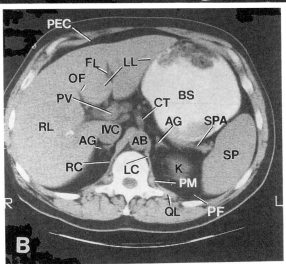

PLATE 40. LV2: right lobe of liver, gallbladder, and spleen: CT scan, oral and intravenous iodinated contrast

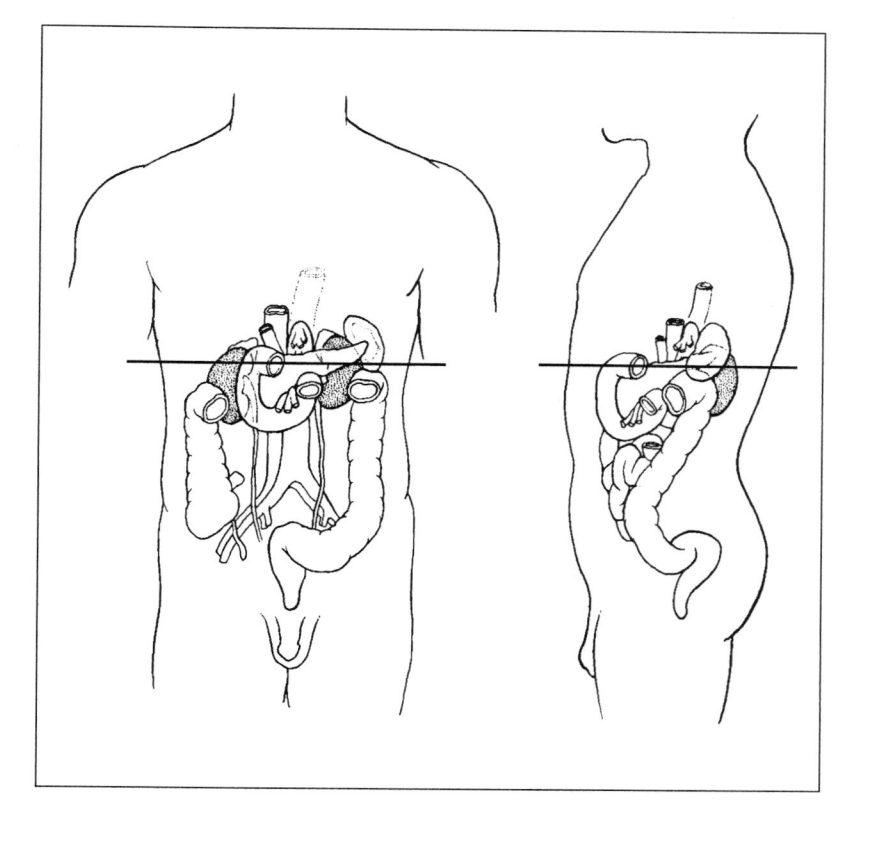

Note

- The surroundings of the abdominal contents at this level include the **2nd lumbar vertebra** (*LV2*), **erector spinae** (*ES*), **psoas major** (*PM*), and **quadratus lumborum** (*QL*), **rib 10** (*R10*), and anterolateral abdominal muscles, including **rectus abdominis** (*RAB*), **external abdominal oblique** (*EO*), **internal abdominal oblique** (*IO*), and **transversus abdominis** (*TA*).
- Between the **right and left lobes of the liver** (*RL, LL*) lies the **gallbladder** (*GB*), and to its left is the **antrum of the stomach** (*PA*).
- The **descending or second part of the duodenum** (*D2*) is lateral and adjacent to the **head of the pancreas** (*P1*). Lying posterior to the **superior mesenteric artery and vein** (*SMA, SMV*) is the **uncinate process** (*UP*) of the pancreas. The **4th part of the duodenum** (*D4*) is seen in **B** as it ends at the **ligament of Treitz** (*TZ*) as the **jejunum** (*J*) begins.
- The **body of the pancreas** (*P2*) extends laterally, posterior to the **body of the stomach** (*BS*), its **tail** (*P3*) reaching to the **spleen** (*SP*).
- The **inferior vena cava** (*IVC*) lies nearly side by side with the **abdominal aorta** (*AB*) as they pass posterior to the **head and body of the pancreas** (*P1, P2*).
- The **superior poles** of both **kidneys** (*K*) and the **renal artery** (*RA*) and **renal vein** (*RV*) are surrounded by copious **perirenal fat** (*PF*).

Clinical Notes

- The superior mesenteric artery is anterior to the left renal vein and may compress it against the aorta, resulting in venous stasis.
- The oblique course of the pancreas usually results in the head, body, and tail being seen on different transaxial images. Imaging of pancreatic disease is currently best performed by CT or diagnostic ultrasound scanning. Fat-suppressed fast MR sequences using oral contrast, if obtained in oblique planes, are very useful in pancreatic imaging.

References G 78-146; N 231-333; RY 271-302

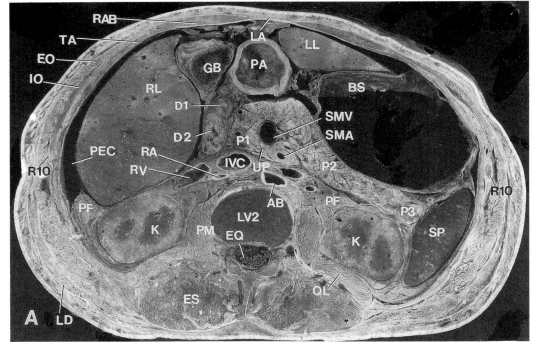

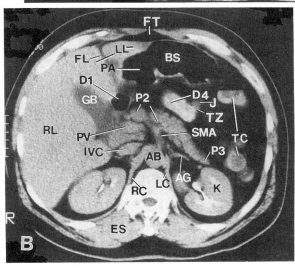

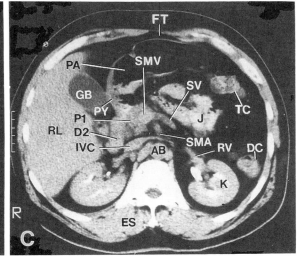

PLATE 41. LV2: right lobe of the liver, hilum of kidneys, and spleen: CT scan, oral and iodinated contrast

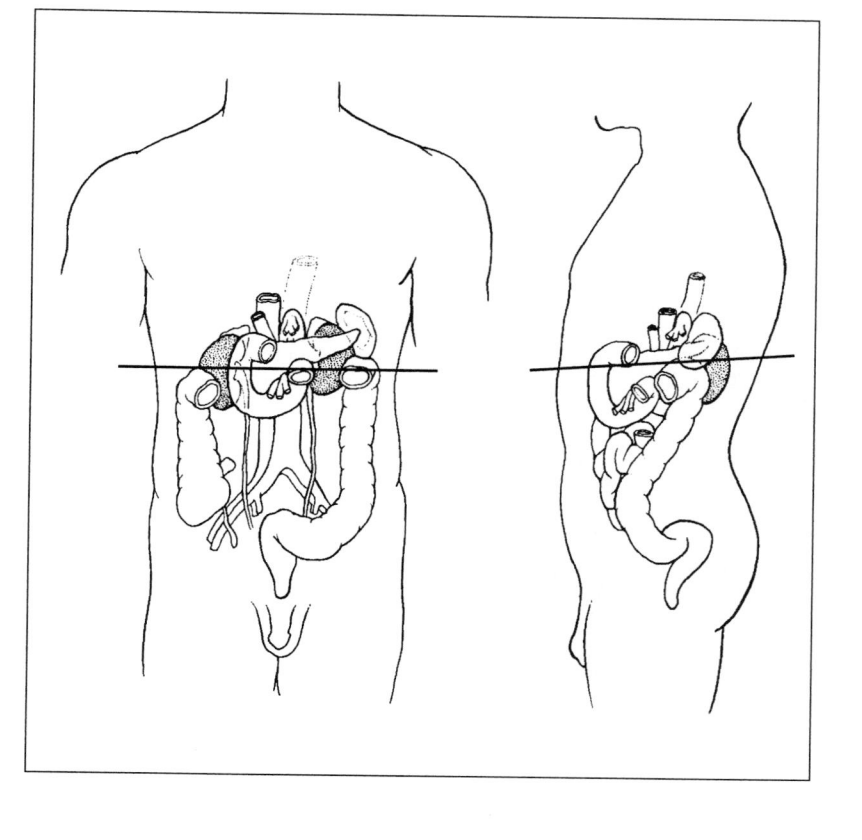

Note

- **A** is inferior to **B**.
- The surroundings of the abdominal contents at this level include the **2nd lumbar vertebra** (*LV2*), **erector spinae** (*ES*), a muscle of the upper limb, **latissimus dorsi** (*LD*), and anterolateral muscles of the abdominal wall: **rectus abdominis** (*RAB*), **external abdominal oblique** (*EO*), **internal abdominal oblique** (*IO*), and **transversus abdominis** (*TA*).
- The **right lobe of the liver** (*RL*) contacts the **transverse colon** (*TC*) to the right of the **antrum of the stomach** (*PA*) at this level.
- The **inferior vena cava** (*IVC*) is nearly side by side with the **abdominal aorta** (*AB*) as both vessels pass posterior to the **uncinate process of the pancreas** (*UP*).
- The **second or descending part of the duodenum** (*D2*) adjoins the **head of the pancreas** (*P1*) laterally and lies between it and two other organs it contacts, i.e., the **right lobe of the liver** (*RL*) and **right kidney** (*K*).
- The left **renal vein** (*RV*) lies anterior to the **renal artery** (*RA*).
- The tip of the lower part of the **spleen** (*SP*) is seen.

Clinical Notes

- The ascending colon, the second part of the duodenum, the pancreas, and the descending colon all lie in contiguity in the anterior pararenal space. Although there is some disagreement about the continuity of space across the midline, this relationship is important in evaluating the contiguous spread of disease.
- Although they are not labeled, the anterolateral muscles of the abdominal wall are clearly seen in **B** on the left side. Compare to the right side of **A**.

References *G* 78-146; **N** 231-333; **RY** 271-302

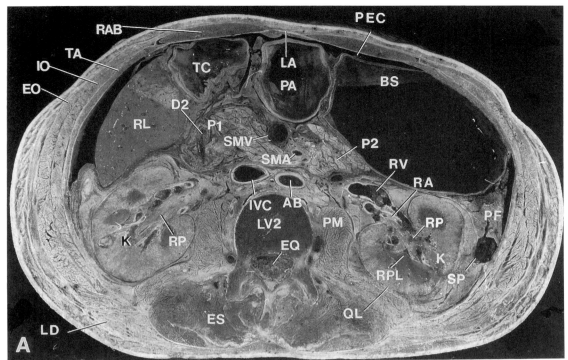

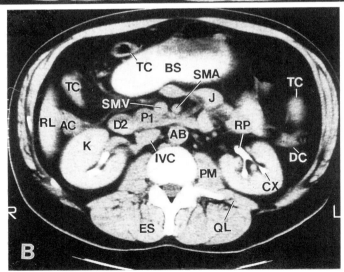

KEY

AB abdominal aorta
AC ascending colon
BS body of stomach
CX renal calyx (minor)
D2 second part of duodenum
DC descending colon

EO external abdominal
   oblique
EQ cauda equina
ES erector spinae
IO internal abdominal oblique
IVC inferior vena cava
J jejunum

K kidney
LA linea alba
LD latissimus dorsi
LV2 body of LV2
P1 head of pancreas
P2 body of pancreas
PA antrum of stomach

PEC peritoneal cavity
PF perirenal fat
PM psoas major
QL quadratus lumborum
RA renal artery
RAB rectus abdominis
RL right lobe of liver

RP renal pelvis
RPL renal papilla
RV renal vein
SMA superior mesenteric
   artery
SMV superior mesenteric vein
SP spleen (lower tip)

TA transversus abdominis
TC transverse colon

PLATE 42. LV3: transverse duodenum, inferior poles of kidneys, and descending colon: CT scan, oral and intravenous iodinated contrast

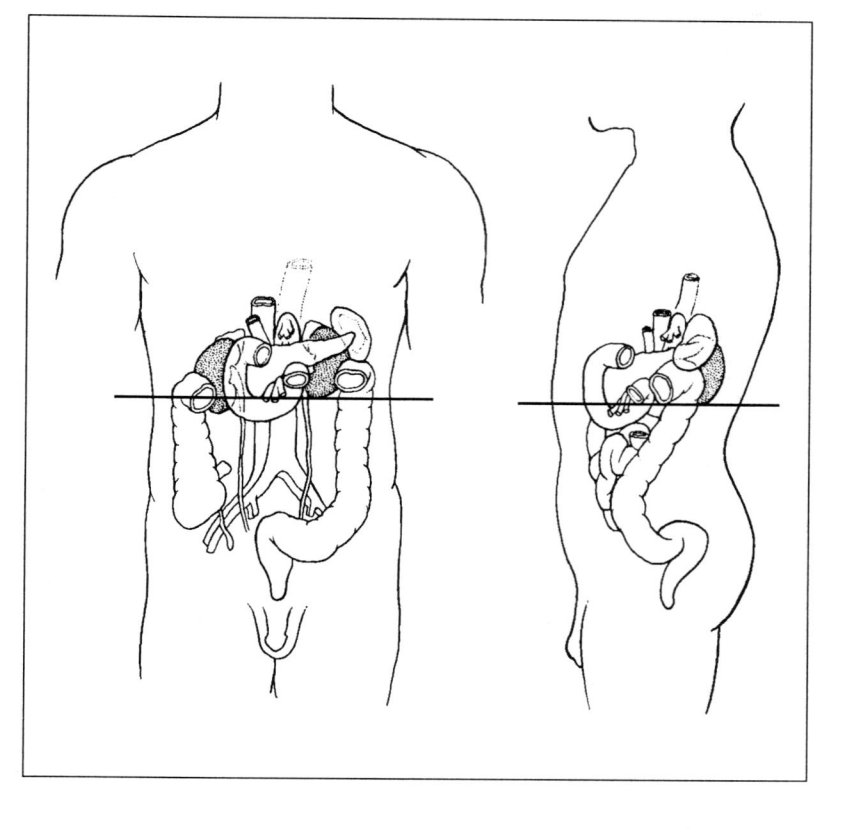

Note

- The surroundings of the abdominal contents at this level include the **3rd lumbar vertebra** (*LV3*), **erector spinae** (*ES*), and anterolateral muscles of the abdominal wall: **rectus abdominis** (*RAB*), **external abdominal oblique** (*EO*), **internal abdominal oblique** (*IO*), and **transversus abdominis** (*TA*).
- The **transverse colon** (*TC*) lies in contact with the surface of the **right kidney** (*K*) and continues towards the contralateral side of the body. The **transverse colon** (*TC*) and **body of stomach** (*BS*) are quite near to the anterior body wall.
- The termination of the **descending part of the duodenum** (*D2*) and the **3rd or transverse part of the duodenum** (*D3*) pass posterior to the **body of the stomach** (*BS*), and anterior to the **abdominal aorta** (*AB*) and the **inferior vena cava** (*IVC*).
- Branches of the **superior mesenteric artery** (*SMA*) and tributaries of the **superior mesenteric vein** (*SMV*) lie within the mesentery seen here between the **body of the stomach** (*BS*) and the **transverse part of the duodenum** (*D3*).
- The **transverse colon** (*TC*) near its termination lies anterior to the **descending colon** (*DC*).
- The **ureters** (*U*) in **A** are seen anterior (right ureter) or anterolateral (left ureter) to the **psoas major muscle** (*PM*).

Clinical Notes

- The superior mesenteric artery lies close to the anterior aspect of the third part of the duodenum. Cachexia can cause the angle between the superior mesenteric artery and the aorta to become even more acute. This in turn causes compression of the third part of the duodenum. The superior mesenteric artery syndrome is a symptom complex that can result.
- The CT scan in **B** has a great deal of fat (black) which acts as natural contrast to the more dense tissues with low water content.
- The anterior location of the stomach allows percutaneous insertion of a feeding tube (gastrostomy).

References G 78-146; N 231-333; RY 271-302

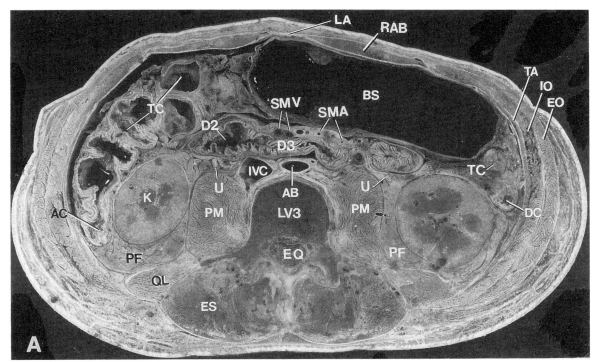

A

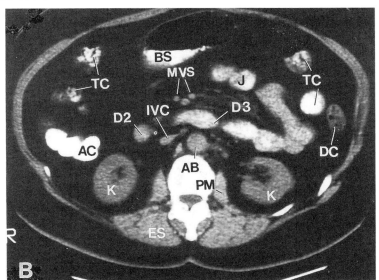

B

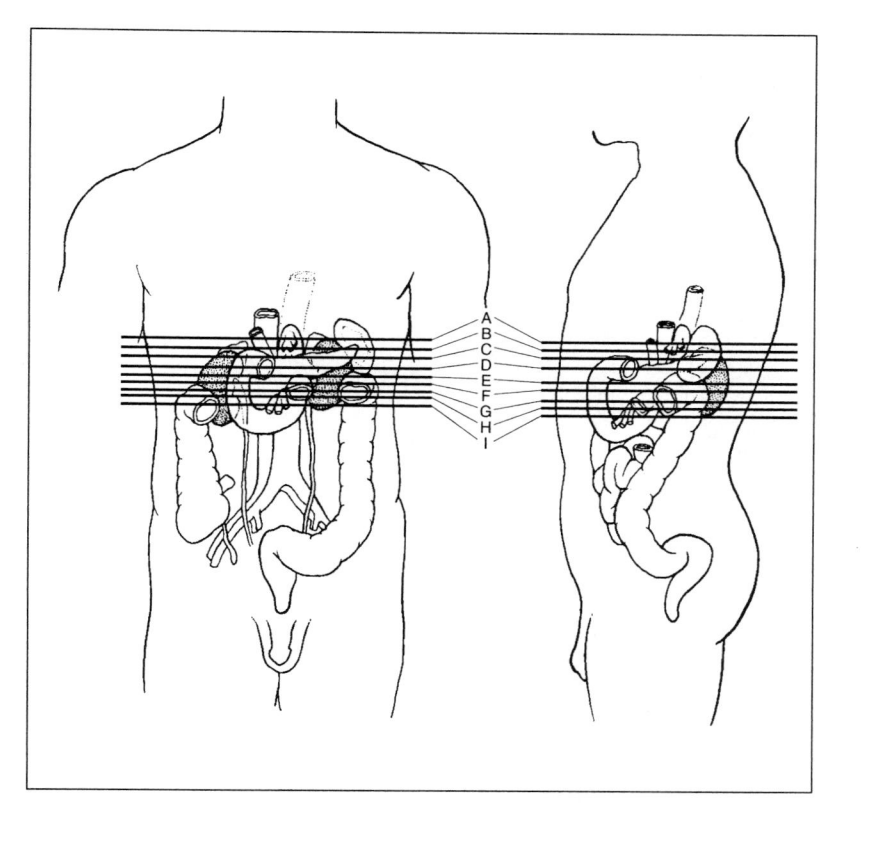

Note

A review of the plate below with images displayed from superior **A** to inferior **I** again emphasizes the usefulness of sequential images and specimens in following the course of structures. The images here fall into the important region just above and below the transpyloric plane (most closely seen at **D**). Concentrating on the **right lobe of the liver** (*RL*) on the right and the **spleen** (*S*) on the left, one sees that both are largest superiorly and that both change from level to level by decreasing in size. The spleen disappears altogether at **D**, whereas the liver continues as far as **I**. Here, as usual, the more superior **left kidney** (*K*) appears first, followed in **B** by the **right kidney** (*K*), both located to the sides of lumbar vertebral bodies. Between the kidneys, anterior to the vertebral bodies are the **inferior vena cava** (*IVC*) to the right and the **abdominal aorta** (*AB*) to the left. The confluence of the **splenic** (*SV*) and **superior mesenteric veins** (*SMV*) is seen in **F**, as they meet to form the **portal vein** (*PV*), seen in **C** and **E**. This occurs anterior to the **inferior vena cava** (*IVC*) and adjacent to the **head of the pancreas** (*P1*).

Clinical Notes

Clearly, observing multiple images allows for a precise analysis of the location and extent of structures or the degree to which pathological processes have involved a region. Review of contiguous slices allows one to evaluate the relationship of lesions to normal structures, such as an abdominal aortic aneurysm to renal artery origins. Further, sequential images of the abdomen are particularly necessary in the clinical setting because of the frequent anatomical variations in the course of longitudinally oriented structures. The delineation of masses is critical both for differential diagnoses and for determining the possible surgical approach.

- In evaluating CT scans, the relationship of the superior mesenteric artery hooking anterior to the left renal vein is important. It allows differentiation from the celiac artery, which is not well seen on these images, and have less than optimal IV contrast density.

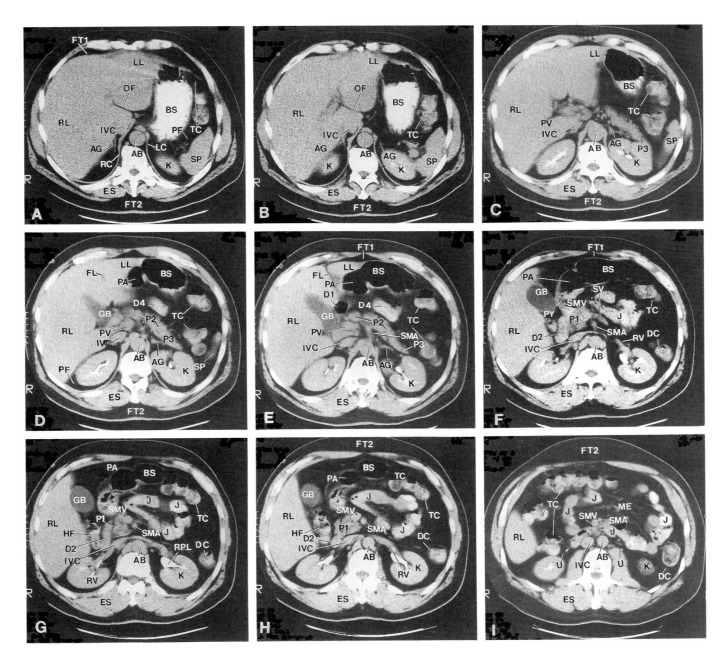

KEY

AB abdominal aorta
AG adrenal gland
BS body of stomach
D1 first part of duodenum
D2 second part of duodenum
D4 fourth part of duodenum

DC descending colon
ES erector spinae
FL falciform ligament
FT1 peritoneal fat
FT2 subcutaneous fat
GB gallbladder
HF hepatic flexure of colon

IVC inferior vena cava
J jejunum
K kidney
LC left crus of diaphragm
LL left lobe of liver
ME mesentery
OF oblique fissure

P1 head of pancreas
P2 body of pancreas
P3 tail of pancreas
PA antrum of stomach
PF perirenal fat
PV portal vein
PY pylorus of stomach

RC right crus of diaphragm
RL right lobe of liver
RPL renal pelvis
RV renal vein
SMA superior mesenteric
  artery
SMV superior mesenteric vein

SP spleen
SV splenic vein
TC transverse colon
U ureter

PLATE 44. Male pelvis, SV1: abdominopelvic junction, iliac fossa, psoas-iliacus junction: T1 MR image

Note

- The surroundings at this level include anterior abdominal musculature—**external abdominal oblique** (*EO*), **internal abdominal oblique** (*IO*), **transversus abdominis** (*TA*), and **rectus abdominis** (*RAB*); the gluteal muscles—**gluteus minimus, medius,** and **maximus** (*GMI, GME, GMA*), **1st sacral vertebra** (*SV1*), and **posterior superior iliac spine** (*PSI*).
- Coils of small bowel, primarily **ileum** (*IL*), sectioned at various angles, occupy much of the major pelvis region between the **ilia of the hip bone** (*ILI*). Posteriorly is part of the **mesentery** (*MS*), supporting the **sigmoid colon** (*SGC*), here sectioned near its termination.
- The iliac fossa is covered by the origin of the **iliacus** (*ILC*), here beginning to merge with the **psoas major** (*PM*) to form iliopsoas. These muscles and other parts of the abdominal wall are covered by **parietal peritoneum** (*PAP*).
- The **femoral nerve** (*FN*) is at the **psoas major** (*PM*) and **iliacus** (*ILC*) junction anteriorly. On the right, the **internal** and **external iliac arteries** (*IA, EA*) and the **common iliac vein** (*CIV*) are medial to **psoas major** (*PM*). The common iliac has divided on the left into the **internal** and **external iliac veins** (*IV, EV*).
- The **sacroiliac joint** (*SIJ*) is seen as well as the **1st pair of anterior sacral foramina** (*ASF*).

Clinical Notes

- Adenopathy is commonly seen along the iliac lymph node chains in the region of the main trunk and branches or tributaries of the common iliac artery and vein.
- The sacroiliac joint can be involved with inflammatory arthropathies such as Reiter's syndrome and ankylosing spondylitis.

References **G** *148-198;* **N** *334-394;* **RY** *303-344*

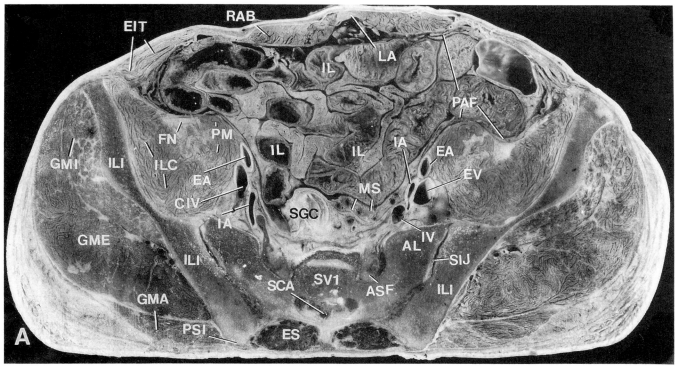

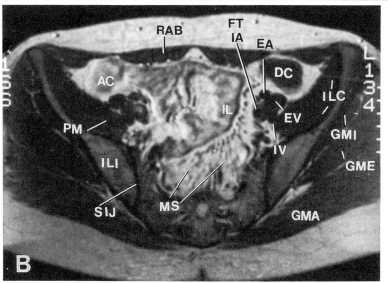

PLATE 45. Male pelvis, SV4: superior aspect of minor pelvis, top of acetabulum, sciatic nerve, piriformis: T1 MR image

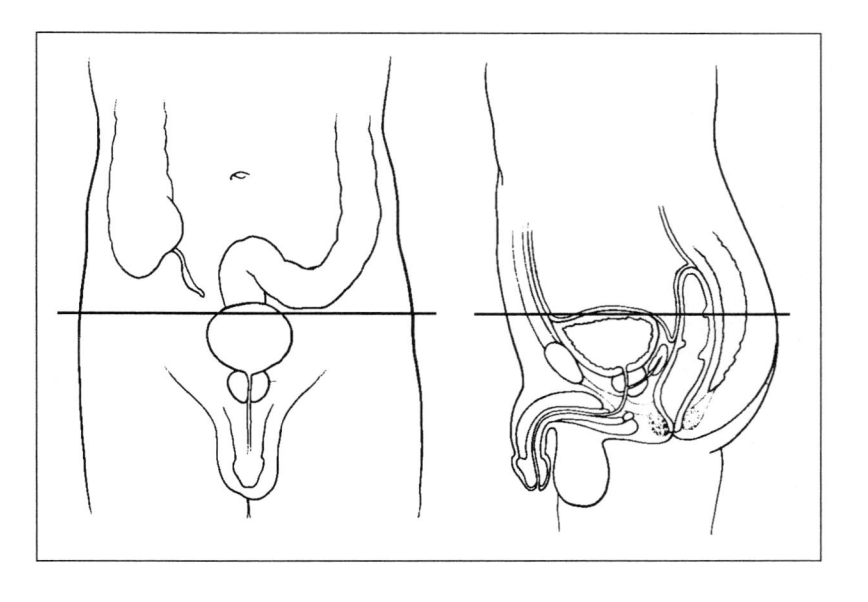

Note

- The surroundings at this level include the inferior part of the **rectus abdominis** (*RAB*) anteriorly, the **sartorius** (*SR*) and **tensor fasciae latae** (*TFL*) anterolaterally, and the gluteal muscles (**gluteus minimus, medius**, and **maximus**—*GMI, GME, GMA*), laterally and posteriorly, and **4th sacral vertebra** (*SV4*) posteriorly.
- Coils of **ileum** (*IL*) occupy much of the minor pelvis between the **iliac bones** (*ILI*). Posteriorly is part of the **mesentery** (*MS*), supporting the **sigmoid colon** (*SGC*), here sectioned near its termination in the **rectum** (*R*).
- The **femoral nerve** (*FN*) lies between the **psoas major** (*PM*) and **iliacus** (*ILC*), and the **external iliac artery** (*EA*) and **external iliac vein** (*EV*) are medial to the **psoas major** (*PM*).
- The **sciatic nerve** (*SN*), **inferior gluteal artery** (*IGA*), and **inferior gluteal vein** (*IGV*), are anterior to the **piriformis** (*PI*). Medial to the **sciatic nerve** (*SN*) and anterior to the **piriformis** (*PI*) is the **pudendal nerve** (*PN*).
- The **sciatic nerve** (*SN*) leaves the pelvis with the **piriformis** (*PI*) through the **greater sciatic foramen** (*black dots*) between the **ilium** (*ILI*) and the sacrum, here represented by the **4th sacral vertebra** (*SV4*).

Clinical Notes

- The sciatic nerve loops behind the posterior column of the acetabulum. This constant relationship is used by radiologists to locate this nerve.
- Metastatic adenopathy or infection that occurs in lymph nodes adjacent to iliac vessels can be seen in MR images.
- The iliacus and psoas muscles will merge on Plate 46 to become the iliopsoas muscle.

References **G** *148-198;* **N** *334-394;* **RY** *303-344*

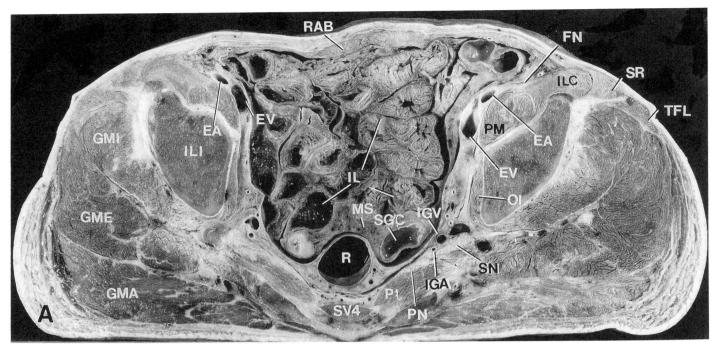

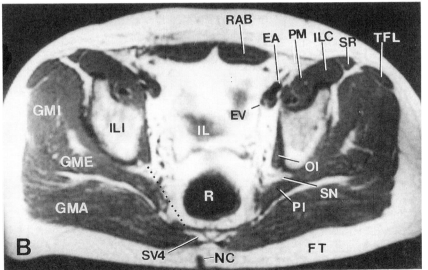

PLATE 46. Male pelvis, coccyx: upper prostate gland, seminal vesicles, acetabulum and greater trochanter: T1 MR image

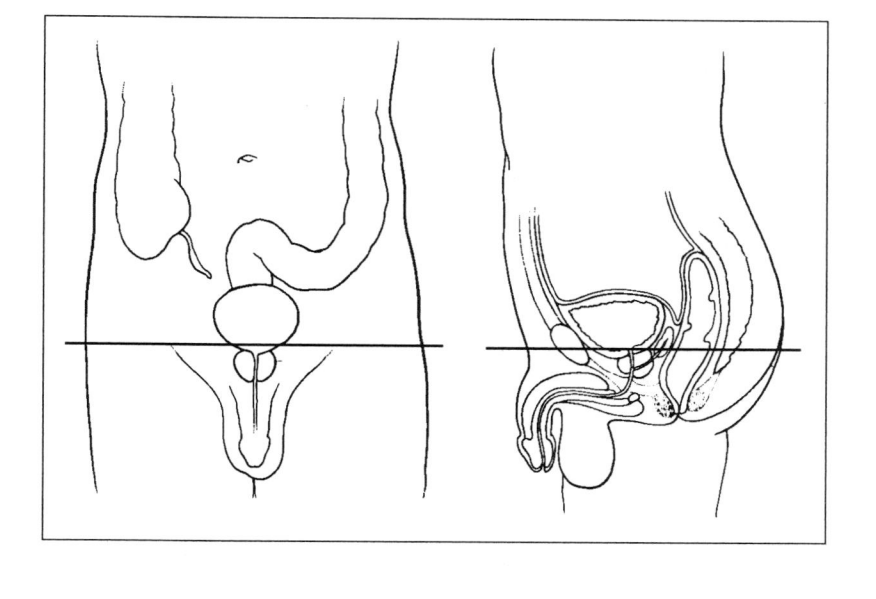

Note

- The specimen in **A** is cut slightly obliquely and lower than **B** and **C**. This explains why the **external iliac artery** and **vein** (*EA, EV*) are seen in **B** and **C** while the **femoral artery** and **vein** (*FA, FV*) are seen in **A**. In living patients, the **urinary bladder** (*BL*) is full, whereas in cadavers, it is usually empty. This causes further variation in the positions of pelvic viscera, which should be kept in mind.
- The surroundings at this level include anteriorly, the **pectineus** (*PEC*), **femoral artery, vein,** and **nerve** (*FA, FV, FN*), and **sartorius** (*SR*); anterolaterally, **rectus femoris** (*RF*) and **tensor fasciae latae** (*TFL*); posteriorly, the **gluteus maximus** (*GMA*) and the **coccyx** (*CCX*).
- The **vas deferens** (*VD*) is seen anteriorly as it passes superiorly in the **spermatic cord** (*SPD*) anterior to the **pectineus** (*PEC*).
- The **femoral nerve** (*FN*) lies anterior to the **iliopsoas** (*IPS*), which is formed from the iliacus and psoas major above this level. The external iliac artery and vein have passed deep to the inguinal ligament above this plane and are now renamed the **femoral artery** and **femoral vein** (*FA, FV*), respectively. They occupy a position between **pectineus** (*PEC*) and **iliopsoas** (*IPS*).
- This section (in **A**) passes through part of the **urinary bladder wall** (*BL*), just posterior to the **pubic symphysis** (*PS*), and reveals the **prostate gland** (*PR*), through which passes the **prostatic urethra** (*PU*). Posterior to the prostate (and slightly superior to it) are the **seminal vesicles** (*SV*). This relationship is well shown in **B** and **C**, **B** being a plane of section above **C**.
- Posterior to both **prostate gland** (*PR*) and **seminal vesicles** (*SV*) is the **rectum** (*R*), and posterior to the rectum is the **coccyx** (*CCX*).
- These midline structures just mentioned are encircled in this plane by muscle, including anterolaterally, the **obturator internus** (*OI*) and posterolaterally, the **iliococcygeus** (*ICG*).
- The **sciatic nerve** (*SN*) lies posteromedial to the **greater trochanter** (*GT*).
- The **gluteus minimus** (*GMI*) attaches anterior to the **gluteus medius** (*GME*) on the **greater trochanter** (*GT*) of the femur.

Clinical Notes

- The acetabulum is a cup-like depression on the lateral side of the hip. It results from fusion in development of ilium, ischium, and pubis. Fractures involving the acetabulum are best understood with multiplanar reconstruction of CT scans. The bones are often described in relation to anterior (iliopubic) or posterior (ilioischial) columns (see also Plate 52).
- At the level of the acetabulum, the external iliac artery becomes the femoral artery and is just superior to the site of femoral venipuncture for injections or blood withdrawals. The close relationship of this artery to the hip joint makes it easy to accidentally enter and contaminate the joint during femoral venipuncture.
- Periprostatic fat, which surrounds the prostate gland, and perirectal fat in the ischiorectal fossa are both loci for tumor infiltration.
- In development, the testes descend along the course of the inguinal canal. Similarly, in indirect abdominal hernias, abdominal organs follow this same course and may be located within or alongside the spermatic cord.

References G *148-198;* ***N*** *334-394;* ***RY*** *303-344*

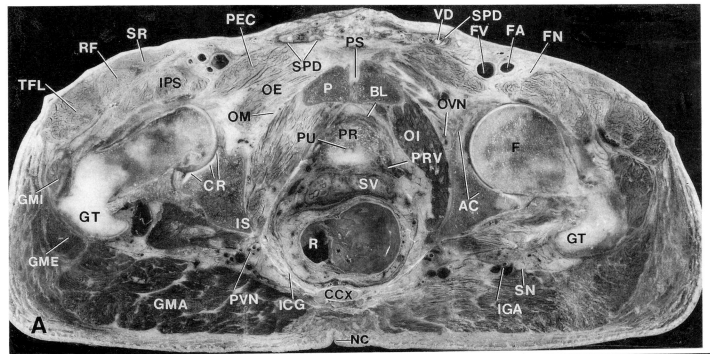

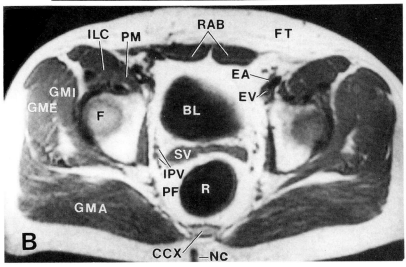

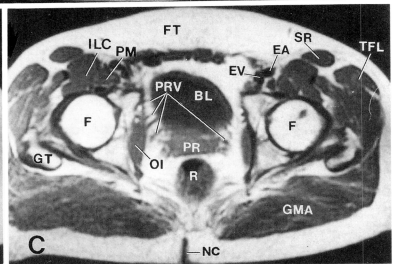

KEY

AC acetabulum	**FA** femoral artery	**ICG** iliococcygeus	**OI** obturator internus	**PR** prostate gland	**RF** rectus femoris
BL urinary bladder	**FN** femoral nerve	**IGA** inferior gluteal artery	**OM** obturator membrane	**PRV** prostatic venous plexus	**SN** sciatic nerve
CCX coccyx	**FT** fat	**ILC** iliacus	**OVN** obturator vessels and	**PS** pubic symphysis	**SPD** spermatic cord
CR hyaline articular cartilage	**FV** femoral vein	**IPS** iliopsoas	nerves	**PU** prostatic urethra	**SR** sartorius
EA external iliac artery	**GMA** gluteus maximus	**IPV** internal pudendal vessels	**P** pubic bone	**PVN** pudendal vessels and	**SV** seminal vesicle
EV external iliac vein	**GME** gluteus medius	**IS** ischium	**PEC** pectineus	nerves	**TFL** tensor fasciae latae
F head of femur	**GMI** gluteus minimus	**NC** natal cleft	**PF** perirectal fat	**R** rectum	**VD** vas deferens
	GT greater trochanter of femur	**OE** obturator externus	**PM** psoas major	**RAB** rectus abdominis	

92

PLATE 47. Male pelvis, coccyx: midprostate gland, greater trochanter, neck of femur: T1 MR image

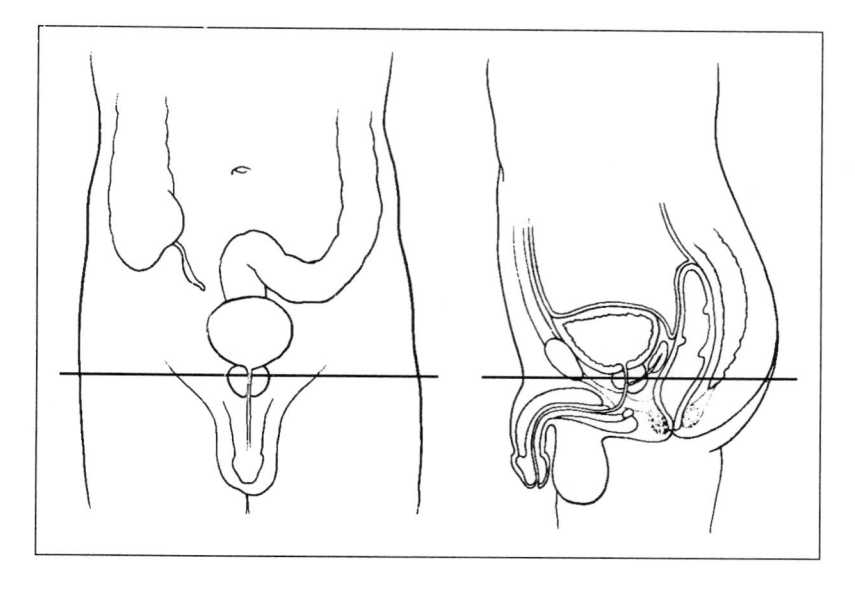

Note

- The surroundings at this level include anteriorly, the **pectineus** (*PEC*), **femoral artery**, **vein,** and **nerve** (*FA, FV, FN*), and **sartorius** (*SR*); anterolaterally, **rectus femoris** (*RF*) and **tensor fasciae latae** (*TFL*) and **vastus lateralis** (*VL*); posteriorly, the **gluteus maximus** (*GMA*) and the **coccyx** (*CCX*).
- The **femoral nerve** (*FN*) lies anterior to the **iliopsoas** (*IPS*). The **femoral vein** (*FV*) lies anterior to **pectineus** (*PEC*), while the **femoral artery** (*FA*) lies between these two muscles.
- The **prostatic venous plexus** (*PVR*) anterior to the **prostate gland** (*PR*) is seen here. The **rectum** (*R*) is posterior to the **prostate gland** (*PR*), and both structures are circled by the **levator ani** (*LEV*).
- The **levator ani** (*LEV*) bounds the **ischiorectal fossa** (*IR*) medially, while the posterior boundary is the **gluteus maximus** (*GMA*), and the lateral boundary is the **obturator internus** (*OI*).
- The **sciatic nerve** (*SN*) lies posterior to the **quadratus femoris** (*QF*) and lateral to the **pudendal vessels** and **nerves** (*PVN*), which lie behind the **ischial tuberosity** (*IT*) at this point.

Clinical Notes

- Prostatic cancer often penetrates the capsule of this gland and extends into the periprostatic fat.
- The ischiorectal fossae communicate with each other over the anococcygeal ligament. Thus, infection in one fossa may spread to the other.
- The obturator foramen formed between pubis and ischial tuberosity is a potential route of communication between pelvic and extrapelvic structures.

References **G** *148-198;* **N** *334-394;* **RY** *303-344*

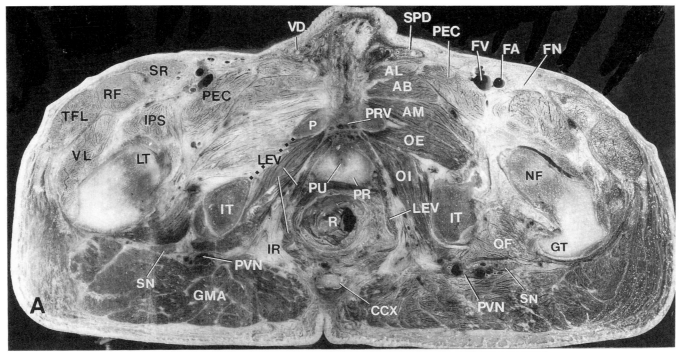

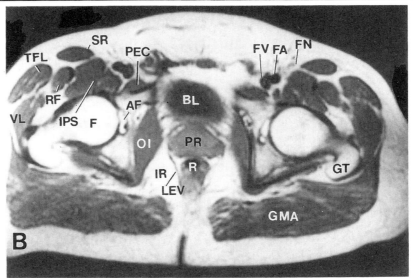

PLATE 48. Male pelvis, anal canal: bulb of penis, ischial tuberosity, shaft of femur: T1 MR image

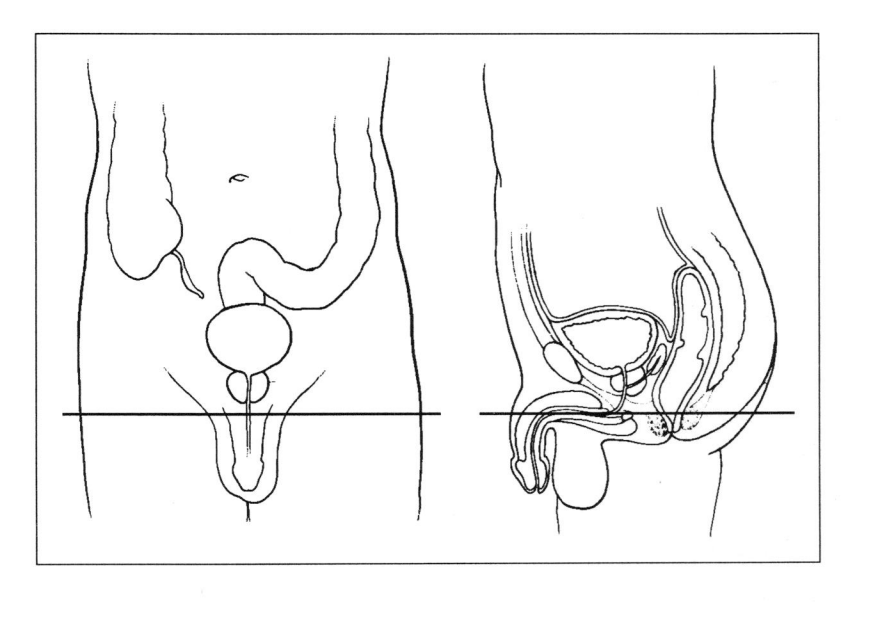

Note

- The surroundings at this level include anteriorly, the male genital organs, **adductor longus** (*AL*), **femoral artery**, **vein,** and **nerve** (*FA, FV, FN*), and **sartorius** (*SR*); anterolaterally, **rectus femoris** (*RF*), **tensor fasciae latae** (*TFL*), and **vastus lateralis** (*VL*); posteriorly, the **gluteus maximus** (*GMA*), and the **natal cleft** (*NC*), on level with the **anal canal** (*A*).
- The **femoral nerve** (*FN*), **femoral vein** (*FV*), and **femoral artery** (*FA*) lie between **adductor longus** (*AL*) and **rectus femoris** (*RF*).
- The erectile tissue of the penis surrounded by the **tunica albuginea** (*ALB*) is seen anteriorly. Towards the dorsum of the penis is the **corpus cavernosum** (*CC*), and ventrally is the (unlabeled) corpus spongiosum, within which lies the spongy **urethra** (*UR*). More posteriorly, between the thighs, one of the two other portions of the **corpus cavernosum** (*CC*) is seen, and in the midline, the **bulb of the penis** (*B*), whose anterior extension becomes the corpus spongiosum, is seen. Also anteriorly, the **pampiniform plexus of veins** (*PX*) is seen in company with the **vas deferens** (*VD*), both of which are contained in the **spermatic cord** (*SPD*).
- The **anal canal** (*A*) is encircled by the **external anal sphincter** (*SPH*), and lies between the two **ischiorectal fossae** (*IR*).
- The **sciatic nerve** (*SN*) lies posterior to the **quadratus femoris** (*QF*) and deep to the **gluteus maximus** (*GMA*).

Clinical Notes

- The pelvis is ideally suited for MR imaging, since intrapelvic organs do not move and there is little motion artifact. Multiplanar imaging allows delimitation of tumor extent in coronal, sagittal, and other oblique orientations as well as in the standard transaxial planes.
- Because they are often multiple and quite variable, many veins are unnamed.
- Due to the insertion of psoas on the lesser trochanter, pathology within it can present as hip pain.

References G 148-198; N 334-394; RY 303-344

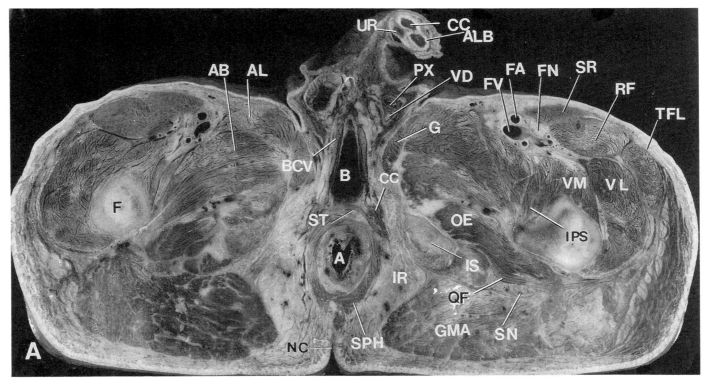

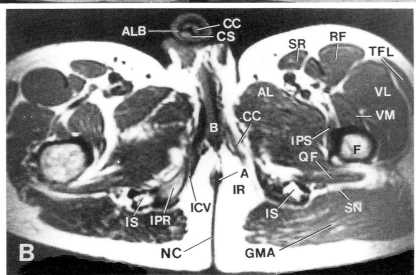

PLATE 49. Female pelvis, coccyx: near superiormost aspect of minor pelvis, top of acetabulum, sciatic nerve: T1 MR image

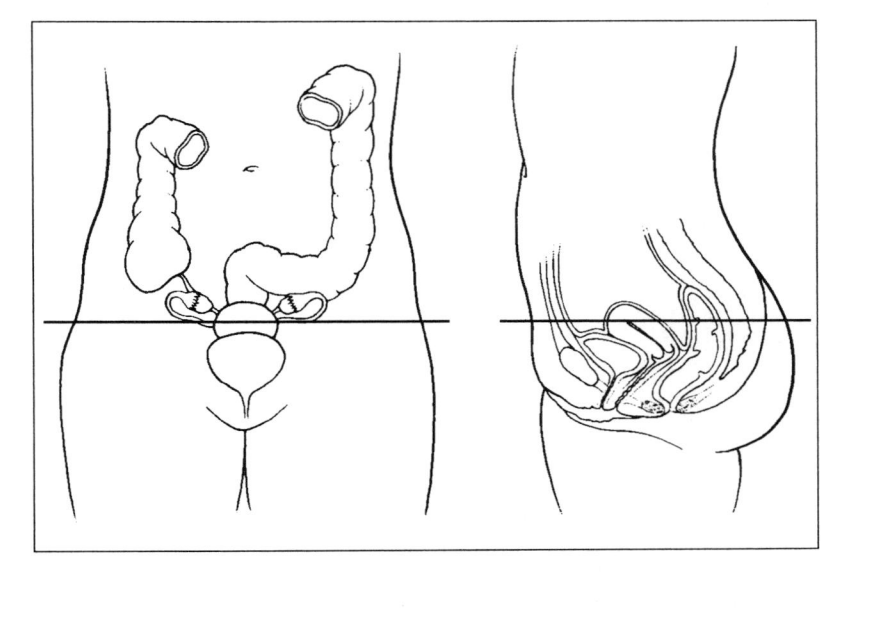

Note

- **A** is cut at a slight angle so that the left side is higher than the right side. **B** is slightly lower than **A** revealing the **vagina** (*VG*). Refer to the previous plates on the male pelvis for many structural similarities, particularly in the region of the hip.
- The surroundings at this level include the inferior part of the **rectus abdominis** (*RAB*) anteriorly, the **iliopsoas** (*IPS*), **sartorius** (*SR*) and **tensor fasciae latae** (*TFL*) anterolaterally, and the gluteal muscles, **gluteus minimus**, **medius**, and **maximus** (*GMI*, *GME*, *GMA*), laterally and posteriorly, and **coccyx** (*CCX*) posteriorly.
- The **ileum** (*IL*) has been displaced from the region above the **body of the uterus** (*UT*) which is covered on both sides by the **broad ligament** (*BL*). Posterior and anterior to the **body of the uterus** (*UT*) the **peritoneal cavity** (*PEC*) is clearly seen. The posterior part of the **peritoneal cavity** (*PEC*) here represents the superior aspect of the **rectouterine pouch of Douglas** (*PD*).
- The course of the **sigmoid colon** (*SG*) from anterolateral to posterior towards the **rectum** (*R*) is seen here.
- The **pudendal vessels and nerves** (*PVN*) lie adjacent to the **ischial spine** (*IS*) just to medial side of the **sciatic nerve** (*SN*).

Clinical Notes

- A most important aspect of staging cervical carcinoma involves the determination of parametrial infiltration, where adenopathy around the obturator internus and iliac lymph node chains may be well demonstrated in MR images.
- The close approximation of the rectum and uterus make it possible to assess the posterior uterus through a bimanual (simultaneous rectal and vaginal) examination.
- The broad band of tissue extending from the uterus to the ovary is the broad ligament, which contains the uterine (fallopian) tubes.
- The low signal (dark) marking the vagina is due to an air tampon placed for localization within it.
- The pouch of Douglas is the most inferior peritoneal recess. It is important as a site of "dropped metastases," ascitic fluid, and infection.

References G 148-198; *N* 334-394; *RY* 303-344

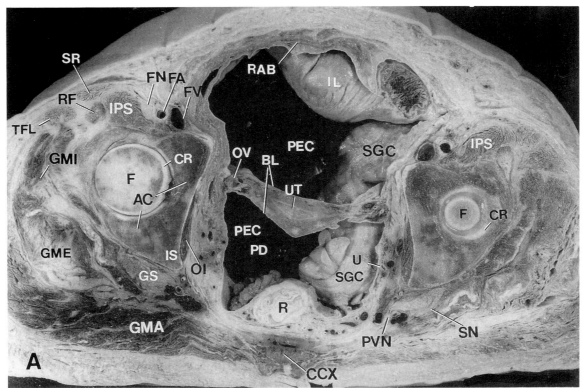

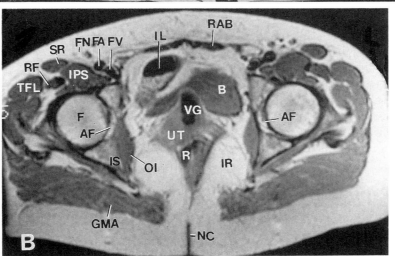

PLATE 50. Female pelvis, coccyx: urinary bladder, obturator foramen, cervix of uterus, and greater trochanter: T1 MR image

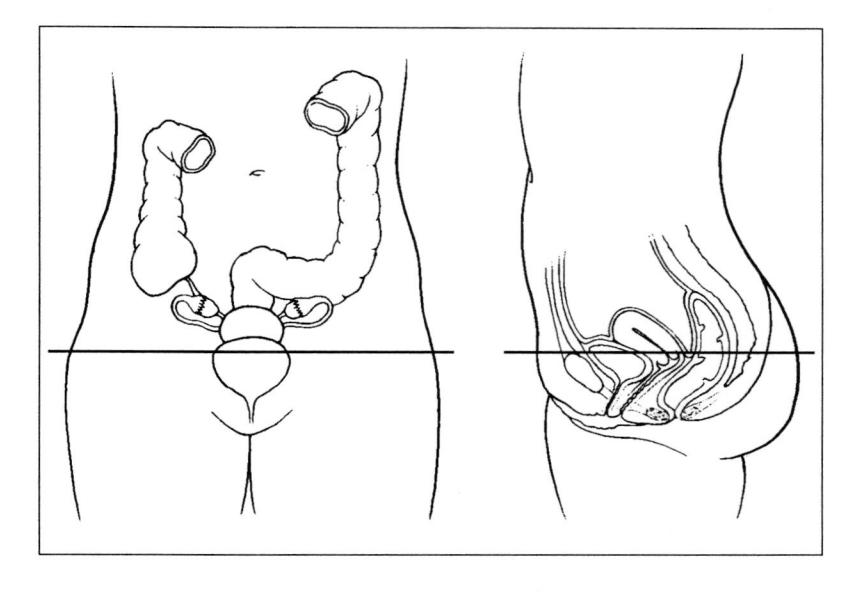

Note

- The surroundings at this level include, anteriorly, the **round ligament of the uterus** (*RL*), **pectineus** (*PEC*), **femoral vein, artery**, and **nerve** (*FV, FA, FN*), and **sartorius** (*SR*); anterolaterally, the **rectus femoris** (*RF*) and **tensor fasciae latae** (*TFL*); posteriorly, the **gluteus maximus** (*GMA*) and the **coccyx** (*CCX*).
- On the lateral side of the pelvic wall in the obturator foramen region, marked by the **obturator vessels** and **nerves** (*OVN*), the **obturator internus** (*OI*) appears just lateral to the **urinary bladder** (*BL*). Behind the bladder is the **cervix of the uterus** (*CX*) and farther posteriorly, the **rectum** (*R*).
- The **pudendal vessels** and **nerves** (*PVN*) appear posterior to the **ischial spine** (*IS*).
- In the MR image in **B**, which is slightly lower, an air tampon marks the position of the **vagina** (*VG*), which at this level is anterior to the **anus** (*A*).
- A more inferior view of the part of the peritoneal cavity seen in the previous plate, the **pouch of Douglas (rectouterine)** (*PD*) appears here. The **rectum** (*R*) in the specimen in **A** is collapsed.

Clinical Notes

- The degree to which infiltration of the parametrium occurs is an important aspect of staging cervical carcinoma.
- The transaxial view of the femoral heads is part of the MR imaging evaluation of avascular necrosis of the femoral head, which further includes coronal images. This diagnosis is based on evaluation of bone marrow, which is particularly well seen on MR images.

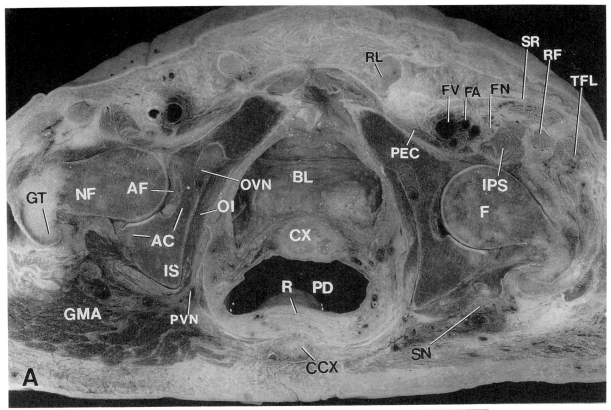

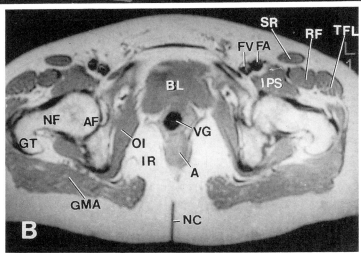

PLATE 51. Female pelvis, rectum near anal canal: ischiopubic rami, crura of clitoris, and superficial perineal space: T1 MR image

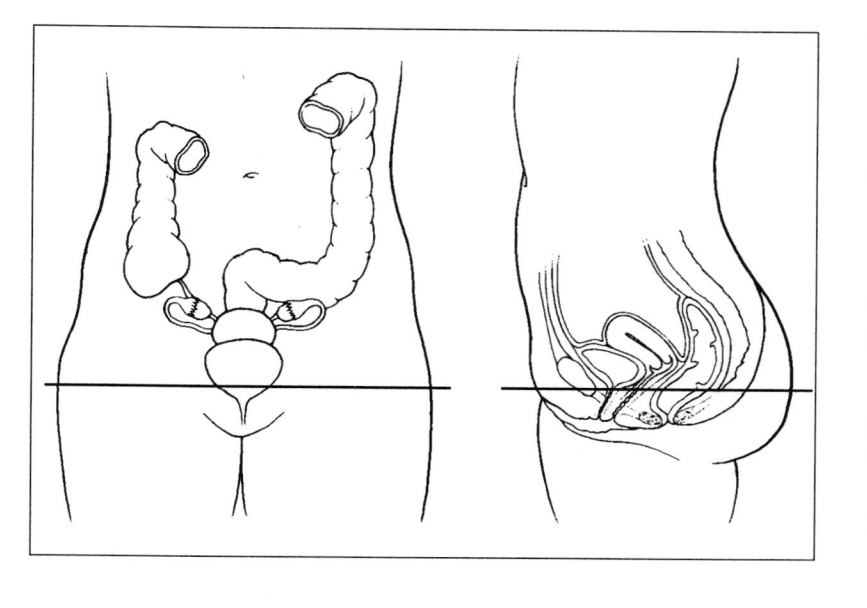

Note

- The surroundings at this level include anteriorly, the **pectineus** (*PEC*), **femoral artery**, **vein**, and **nerve** (*FA, FV, VN*), and **sartorius** (*SR*); anterolaterally, **rectus femoris** (*RF*) and **tensor fasciae latae** (*TFL*); posteriorly the **gluteus maximus** (*GMA*), and the **rectum** (*R*) at the anorectal sling portion of the **levator ani** (*LEV*).
- The **crura of the clitoris** (*CR*) flank the **urethral orifice** (*UR*), which here lies close to the neck of the urinary bladder. The orifice is dilated from emplacement of a catheter into this older patient before her death. Behind it lies the crescentrically shaped cavity of the **vagina** (*VG*). Extending from the **crura of the clitoris** (*CR*) are the **ischiocavernosi** (*ICV*).
- Encircling the posterior side of the **rectum** (*R*) is the **levator ani** (*LEV*).
- The **shaft of the femur** (*F*) with accompanying vasti muscles, including **vastus lateralis** and **medialis** (*VL, VM*) is seen.

Clinical Notes

- The narrowest dimension of the birth canal is measured as the distance between the ischial tuberosities, which are seen bilaterally in **B**.
- On the more caudal MR image seen here, the anus has terminated and is not seen.

*References **G** 148-198; **N** 334-394; **RY** 303-344*

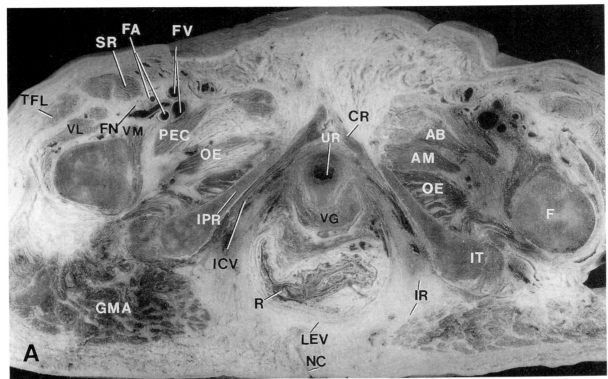

A

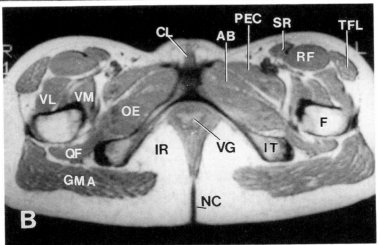

B

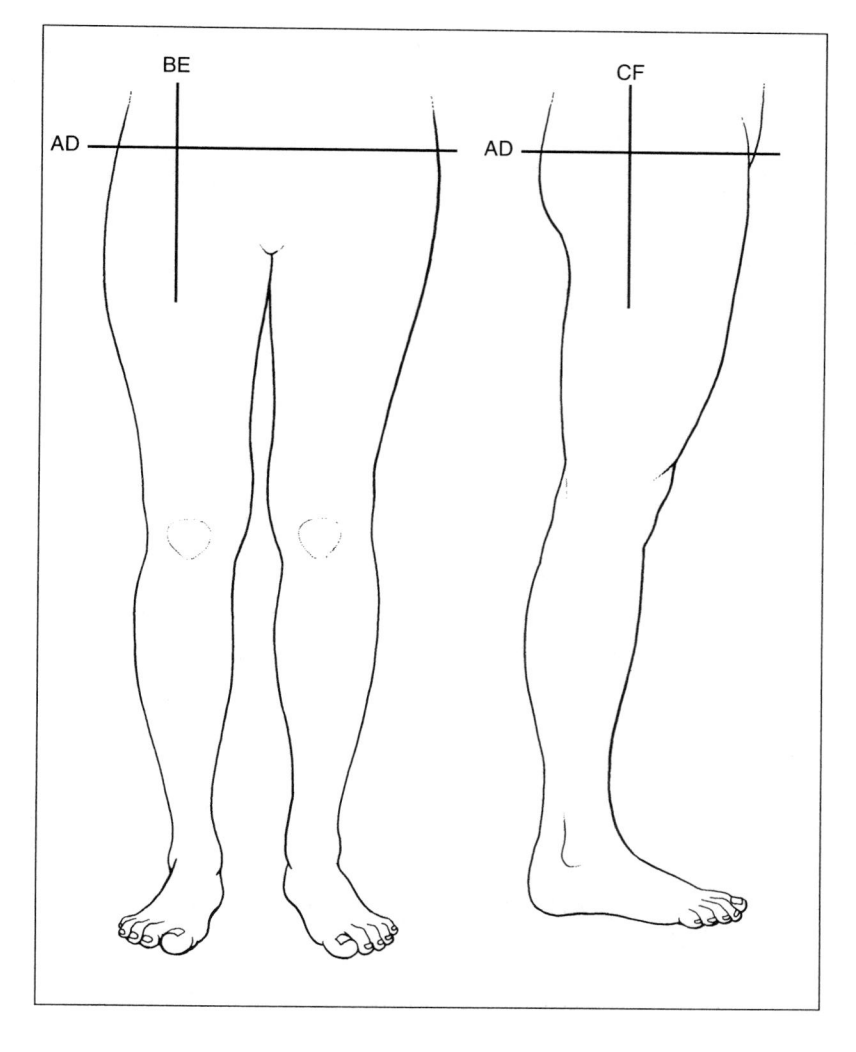

Note

- The transaxial section in **A** passes through the **greater trochanter** (*GT*) and **neck** (*NF*) and **head** (*HF*) of the femur, whose shape conforms to a cup-like structure on the lateral surface of the hip bone, the **acetabulum** (*AC*), also seen in the sagittal **B** and **E** and coronal **C** and **F** views.
- From medial to lateral and directly anterior to the hip joint are the **femoral vein** and **artery** (*FV, FA*) and the **femoral nerve** (*FN*).
- The muscles anterior and lateral to the hip joint include the **iliopsoas** (*IPS*), **sartorius** (*SR*), **rectus femoris** (*RF*), and **tensor fasciae latae** (*TFL*). The disposition of the **iliopsoas** (*IPS*) is further seen in the sagittal plane in **B, E,** and **F** as this muscle passes from its iliac and lumbar attachments to its attachment at the lesser trochanter.
- In **A**, the **gluteus maximus** (*GMA*) appears as the principal posterior muscle component. This is also apparent in **B** and **E,** where, in addition, deep to the **gluteus maximus** (*GMA*) and superficial to **obturator internus** (*OI*) and **quadratus femoris** (*QF*), the **sciatic nerve** *SN* is seen. The location of this nerve posterior or superficial to the **obturator internus** (*OI*) is also seen in the transaxial sections **A** and **B**.
- The view in **C** and **F** displays the hip joint's position relative to male pelvic organs, the **prostate** (*PR*) and **bladder** (*BL*), and **F** presents the disposition of the various muscles around the hip joint especially clearly.
- As you study the views of the muscles around joints, notice that their positions suggest their function. Here, **iliopsoas** (*IPS*) is clearly a flexor of the thigh, whereas the **gluteus maximus** (*GMA*) is an extensor of the thigh. Similarly, the **gluteus medius** (*GME*) and **gluteus minimus** (*GMI*) from their appearance lateral to the hip joint, are thigh abductors, whereas the **pectineus** (*PEC*) is a thigh adductor.

Clinical Notes

- In performing a femoral venipuncture, the pulsating femoral artery is palpated in the groin, and the needle is inserted medial to it.
- On T1 MR images the low signal (dark) of cortical bone is not separated from low-signal (dark) cartilage.
- The acetabulum develops by fusion in the development of ilium, ischium, and pubis. These bones contribute named portions of the acetabulum, fracture of which is best understood with multiplanar reconstruction (MPR) CT. The bones are often described in relation to anterior (iliopubic) or posterior (ilioischial) columns.

References **G** 4-34, 4-51; **N** 457-461, 474; **RY** 418-419; 426-427

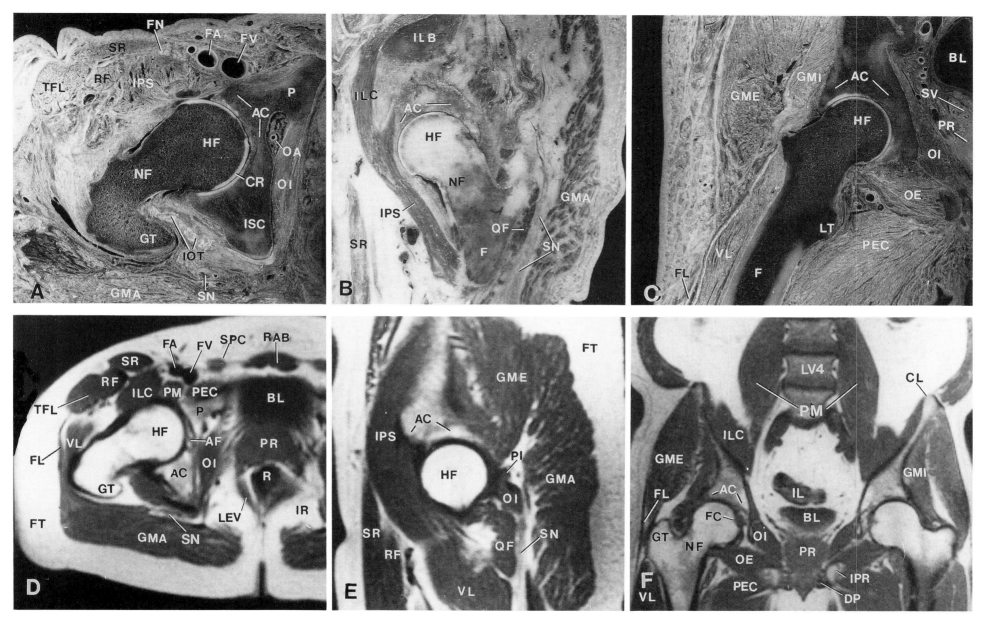

KEY

AC acetabulum	**FC** fovea	**HF** head of femur	**LEV** levator ani	**PI** piriformis	**SR** sartorius
AF acetabular fat	**FL** fascia lata	**IL** ileum	**LT** lesser trochanter	**PM** psoas major	**SV** seminal vesicle
BL urinary bladder	**FN** femoral nerve	**ILB** ilium	**LV4** lumbar vertebra 4	**PR** prostate gland	**TFL** tensor fasciae latae
CL crest of ilium	**FT** subcutaneous fat	**ILC** iliacus	**NF** neck of femur	**QF** quadratus femoris	**VL** vastus lateralis
CR hyaline articular cartilage	**FV** femoral vein	**IOT** obturator internus tendon	**OA** obturator artery	**R** rectum	
DP deep perineal pouch	**GMA** gluteus maximus	**IPR** ischiopubic ramus	**OE** obturator externus	**RAB** rectus abdominis	
F shaft of femur	**GME** gluteus medius	**IPS** iliopsoas	**OI** obturator internus	**RF** rectus femoris	
FA femoral artery	**GMI** gluteus minimus	**IR** ischiorectal fossa	**P** pubic bone	**SN** sciatic nerve	
	GT greater trochanter	**ISC** ischium	**PEC** pectineus	**SPC** spermatic cord	

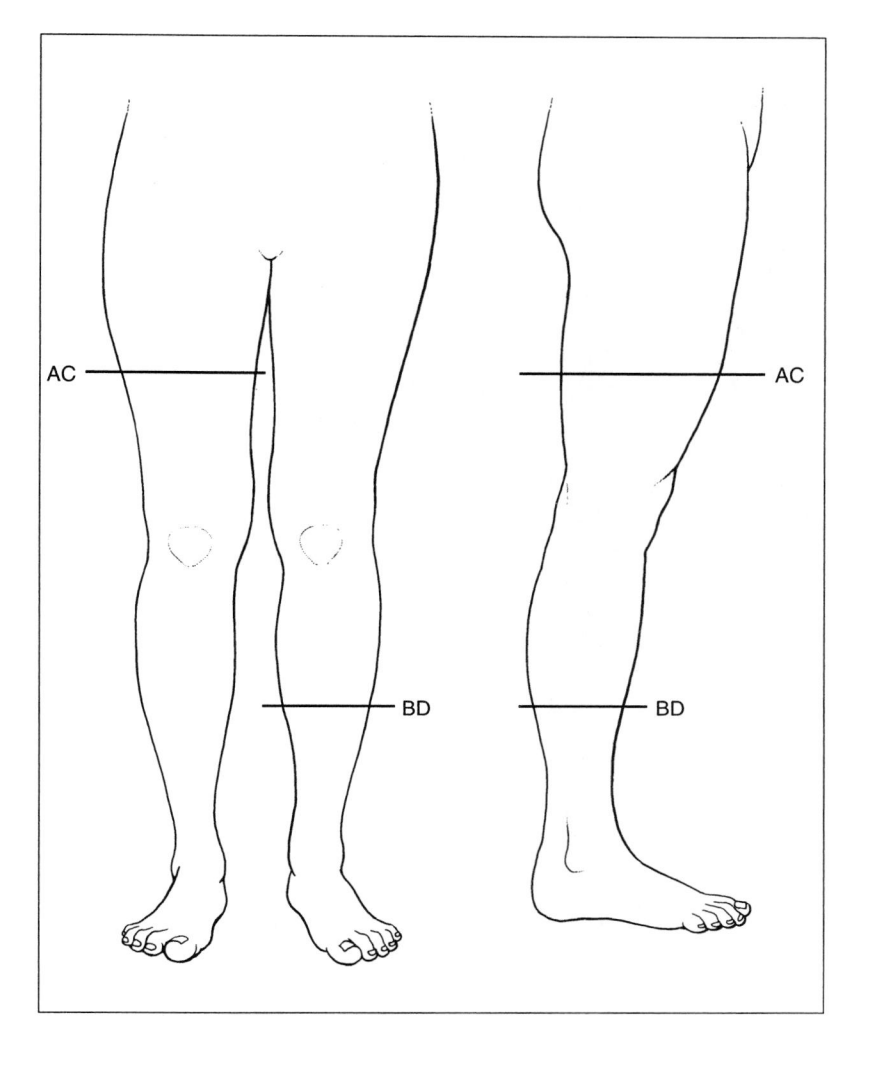

Note

- The compartmentalization of the thigh into anterior, medial, and posterior compartments, and the leg into anterior, lateral, and posterior compartments is indicated in Figures 2B, 16, and 17.

Thigh: A, C

- The anterior musculature, including the **rectus femoris** (RF), **vastus medialis** (VM), **vastus lateralis** (VL), and **vastus intermedius** (VIM), wrap around most of the femur, leaving only the region of the **linea aspera** (LA) for the attachment of other muscles.
- The subsartorial canal, whose boundaries are the **adductor longus** (AL) posteriorly, **vastus medialis** (VM) laterally, and **sartorius** (SR) medially, contains the **femoral artery** (FA), **femoral vein** (FV), and the **saphenous nerve** (SPN).
- The **great or long saphenous vein** (LSV), embedded in fatty subcutaneous tissue, lies medial to the **adductor longus** (AL).
- The **sciatic nerve** (SN) lying on the anterior surface of the long head of the **biceps femoris** (BF) is the major nerve component of the posterior compartment of the thigh.

Leg: B, D

- **D** is slightly rotated counterclockwise to **B**.
- The **tibia** (TI) or bone of the medial side of the leg is subcutaneous, while the **fibula** (FI), laterally, is covered by a thick layer of muscle.
- The **posterior tibial artery and vein** (PTA, PTV) and the accompanying **tibial nerve** (TN) lie in the posterior compartment behind the **tibialis posterior** (TP), which itself rests on the **interosseous membrane** (IOM).
- The **anterior tibial artery and vein** (ATA, ATV) and the accompanying **deep peroneal nerve** (DPN) lie just anterior to the **interosseous membrane** (IOM).
- The lateral compartment of the leg, which is as much anterior as it is lateral, contains two muscles, the **peroneus longus** (PL) and deep to it, the **peroneus brevis** (PB).

Clinical Notes

- MR imaging is the best modality for defining soft tissue masses in the extremities.
- Since the anterior compartment muscles "wrap around" it, it is difficult to palpate the shaft of the femur.
- In the leg, swelling confined to a specific compartment created by fascial planes, may cause ischemia and clinical "compartment syndrome."
- Popliteal cysts adjacent to the lateral head of the gastrocnemius muscles can be seen on MR images, although routine x-ray arthrography and diagnostic ultrasound will also show this pathological condition.

References Thigh—**G** 5-15 to 5-37, 5-52 A, B, C; **N** 461-465, 475; **RY** 426, 430, 468. **Leg**—**G** 5-97 A, B; **N** 482, 491; **RY** 431-436; 469

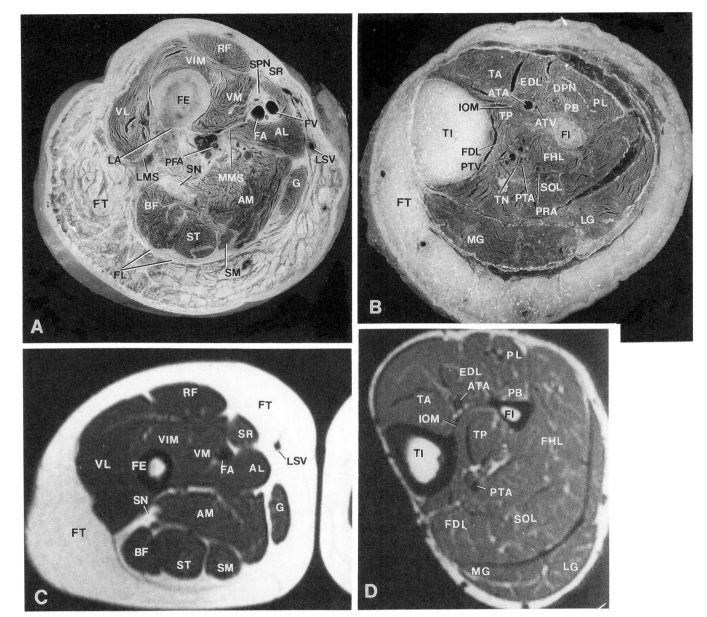

KEY

AL adductor longus
AM adductor magnus
ATA anterior tibial artery
ATV anterior tibial vein
BF biceps femoris
DPN deep peroneal nerve
EDL extensor digitorum longus

FA femoral artery
FDL flexor digitorum longus
FE shaft of femur
FHL flexor hallucis longus
FI fibula
FL fascia lata
FT subcutaneous fat
FV femoral vein
G gracilis

IOM interosseous membrane
LA linea aspera
LG lateral head, gastrocnemius
LMS lateral intermuscular septum
LSV long saphenous vein
MG medial head, gastrocnemius

MMS medial intermuscular septum
PB peroneus brevis
PFA profunda femoris artery
PL peroneus longus
PRA peroneal artery
PTA posterior tibial artery
PTV posterior tibial vein
RF rectus femoris

SM semimembranosus
SN sciatic nerve
SOL soleus
SPN saphenous nerve
SR sartorius
ST semitendinosus
TA tibialis anterior
TI tibia
TN tibial nerve

TP tibialis posterior
VIM vastus intermedius
VL vastus lateralis
VM vastus medialis

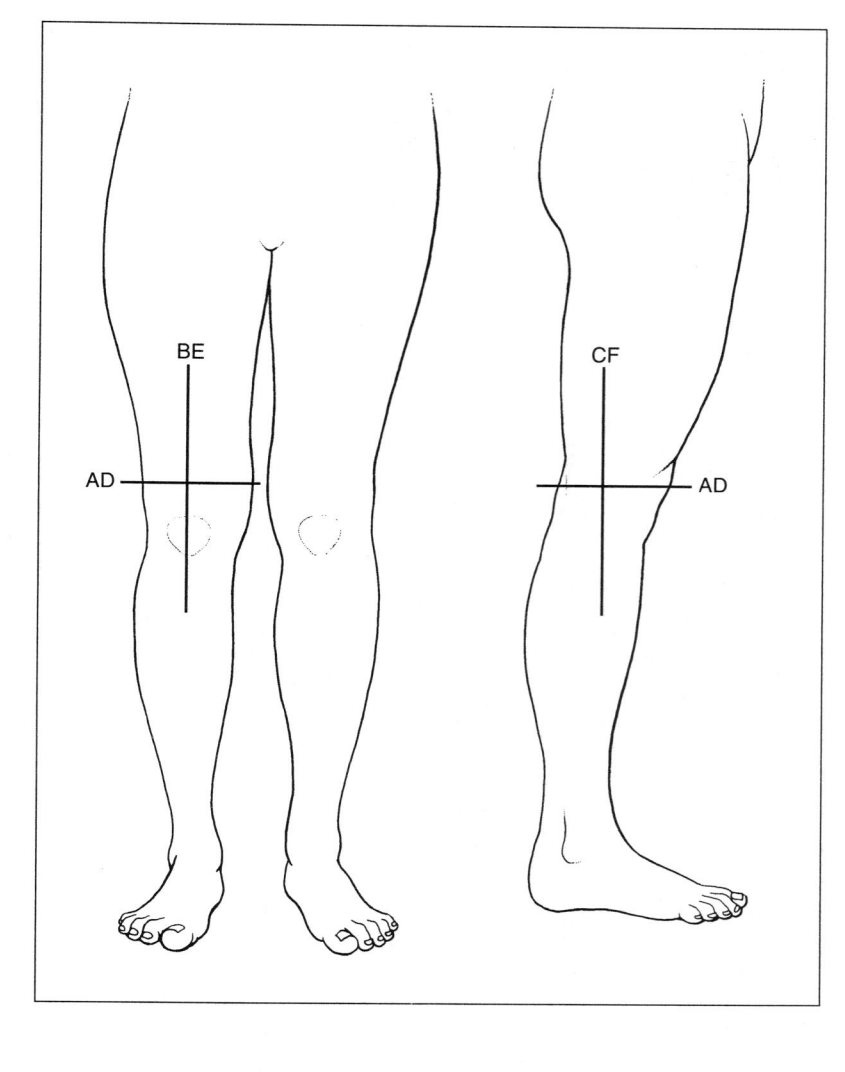

Note

- Musculotendinous structures surrounding the knee and seen in **A** include: anterolaterally and anteromedially tendons of **vastus lateralis** (VL) and **vastus medialis** (VM); posterolaterally, **biceps femoris** (BF); posteromedially, **semimembranosus** (SM), **semitendinosus** (ST), **gracilis** (G), and **sartorius** (SR).
- The expanded distal end of the **femur** (FE) is seen in **A**, in the popliteal region posterior to it are the **popliteal artery** (PA), **popliteal vein** (PV), **tibial nerve** (TN), and **common peroneal nerve** (PN).
- In **B** and **C**, the course and positions of the **anterior cruciate** (AP) and **posterior cruciate** (PC) ligaments are seen.
- The **hyaline articular cartilage** (CR) (**A,B,C**) associated with the patella and other parts of the knee joint is normally, as here, quite thick.
- In **C**, the deep attachment of the **medial collateral ligament** (MCL) to the **medial meniscus** (MM), called the coronoid ligament, is more posterior and not seen on this section.
- Note the "slice of pie" shape of the **medial** and **lateral menisci** (LM, MM) on the coronal image.

Clinical Notes

- Although overall morphology is best seen on these T1 images, a variety of specific pulse sequences with acronyms like GRASS produce images that specifically accentuate different tissues such as meniscal cartilage. Meniscal tears can usually be diagnosed by weighted spin echo GRASS imaging.
- Low-signal (dark) tendons blend with low-signal cortical bone.
- The normal high (bright) signal from bone marrow can be decreased in the presence of bone bruise which is defined as a traumatic lesion, possibly microtrabecular fracture, without plain radiographic findings.
- Because its oblique course is more nearly oriented in the true sagittal plane, the posterior cruciate is usually completely seen on a single image, while the anterior cruciate is not.

References G 5-55 to 5-73; **N** 476-480; **RY** 432, 469

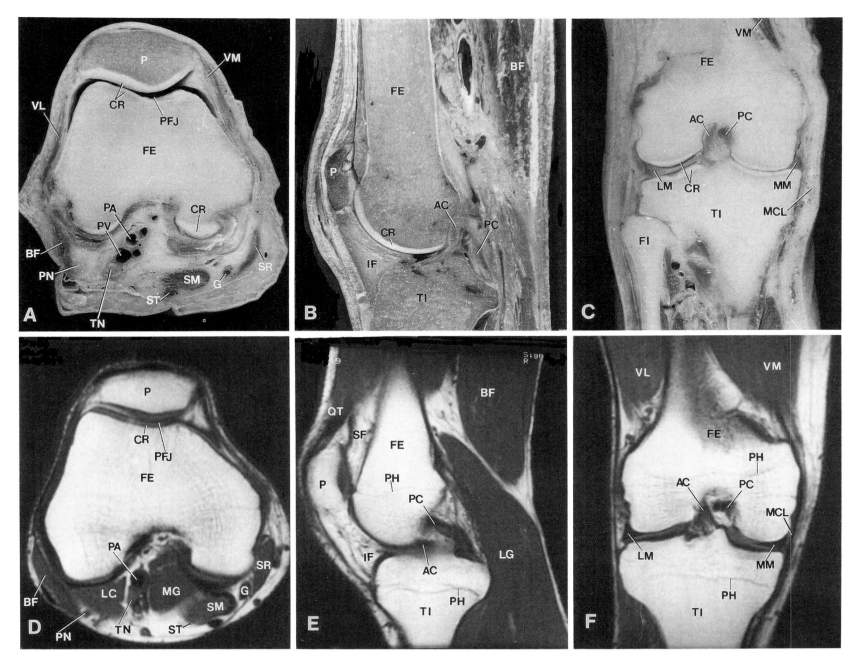

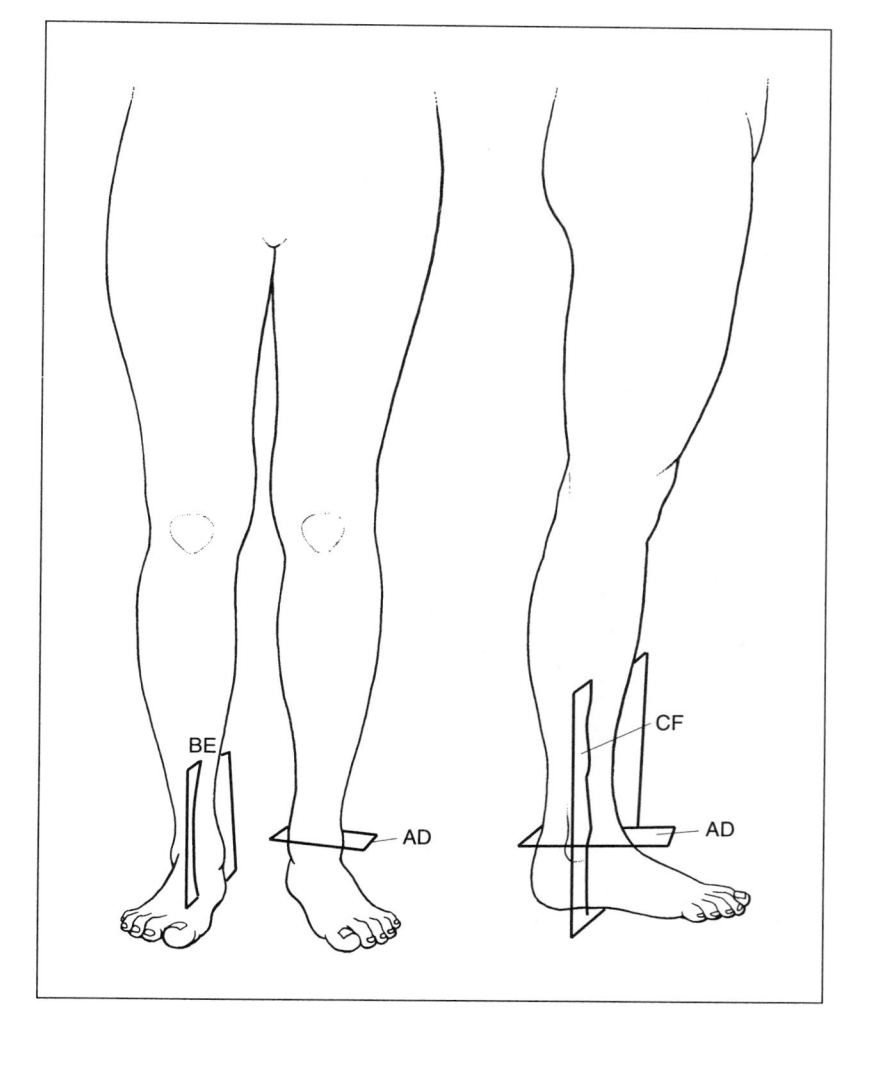

Note

- The coronal views (**C** and **F**) reveal bones and articular surfaces participating in the **ankle joint** (**talocrural**, or in clinical use, **tibiotalar**) (*AJ*). These bones are the superior, medial, and lateral aspects of the **talus** (*TAL*), with the lateral side of the **medial malleolus** (*MM*) and the medial side of the **lateral malleolus** (*LM*).
- The sagittal views (**B** and **E**) and coronal (**C** and **F**) views reveal bones and articular surfaces of the **talus** (*TAL*) and **calcaneus** (*CAL*) participating in the **subtalar joint** (*STJ2*). In **B** and **E**, this joint is seen to be composed of **anterior subtalar** (*STJ1*) and **posterior subtalar** (*STJ2*) parts.
- The sagittal views (**B** and **E**) also show the **talonavicular joint** (*TNJ*) between the **talus** (*TAL*) and **navicular** (*NV*). Lateral to this latter joint, out of the plane of section in **B**, but appearing in the MR image in **E**, is the **calcaneocuboid joint** (*CCJ*). Together, these two joints form the midtarsal joint.
- The sagittal views (**B** and **E**) show the **calcaneus** (*CAL*), **navicular** (*NV*), **2nd cuneiform** (*CU2*) and **2nd metatarsal** (*MT2*). With the 1st cuneiform and 1st metatarsal, which are out of the plane of section here, these bones form a medial longitudinal plantar arch.
- The anterior and posterior nerve, vessel, and muscle tendon relationships are best seen in transaxial sections **A** and **D**. Here, muscles that extend (dorsiflex) the ankle joint or toes (**extensor hallucis longus** [*EHL*], **extensor digitorum longus** [*EDL*], and **tibialis anterior** [*TA*]) lie anterior to the **intermalleolar plane** (*black line*). Flexor tendons lie posterior to this plane. Most posteriorly, the gastrocnemius and part of the soleus (out of this plane) insert together as the **tendo calcaneus (Achilles tendon)** (*TC*); behind the **medial malleolus** (*MM*) is the **tibialis posterior** (*TP*), and behind it the **flexor digitorum longus** (*FDL*) and **flexor hallucis longus** (*FHL*) retained in position by the **flexor retinaculum** (*FR*); behind the **lateral malleolus** (*LM*) lie the **peroneus longus** and **brevis** (*PL, PB*), retained in position by the **peroneal retinaculum** (*PR*).
- Observation of sagittal sections (**B** and **E**) reveals that the posterior muscles **gastrocnemius** and **soleus** (*GA, SO*) would tend to be stronger flexors of the **ankle joint** (*AJ*) than the other posterior muscles, which act more strongly: (a) in flexion of the tarsometatarsal joints represented here by the **cubometatarsal joint** (*CMJ*); (b) in flexion of the metacarpophalangeal joints, represented here by the **2nd metacarpophalangeal joint** (*MPJ*); and (c) in inversion-eversion at the **subtalar** (*STJ*), **talonavicular** (*TNJ*), and **calcaneocuboid joints** (*CCJ*).

Clinical Notes

- The interosseous ligament passes through the sinus tarsi, an oblique space between talus and calcaneus filled with fat.
- On T1 sequences, cortex and cartilage both have a low (dark) signal.
- Avascular necrosis of the talus, appears as a change in the normal marrow signal in MRI.

References G 5-100 to 5-130; N 494-499; RY 461-465

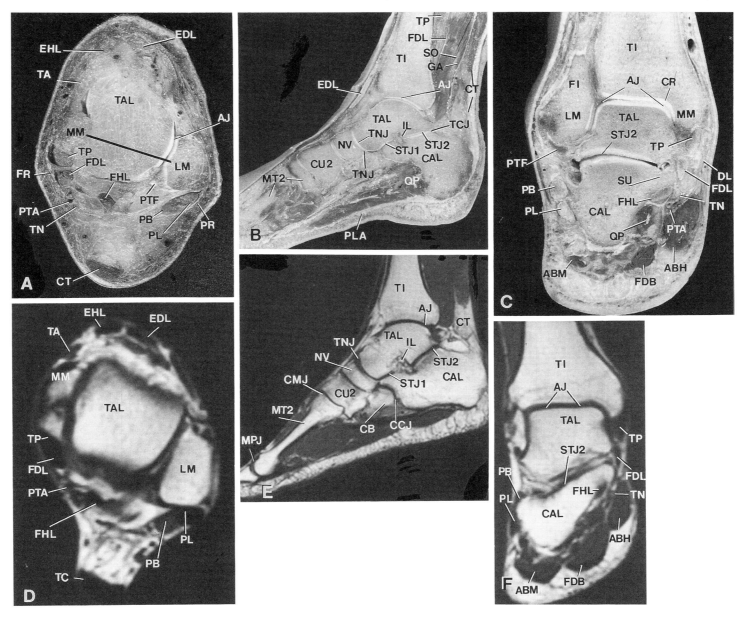

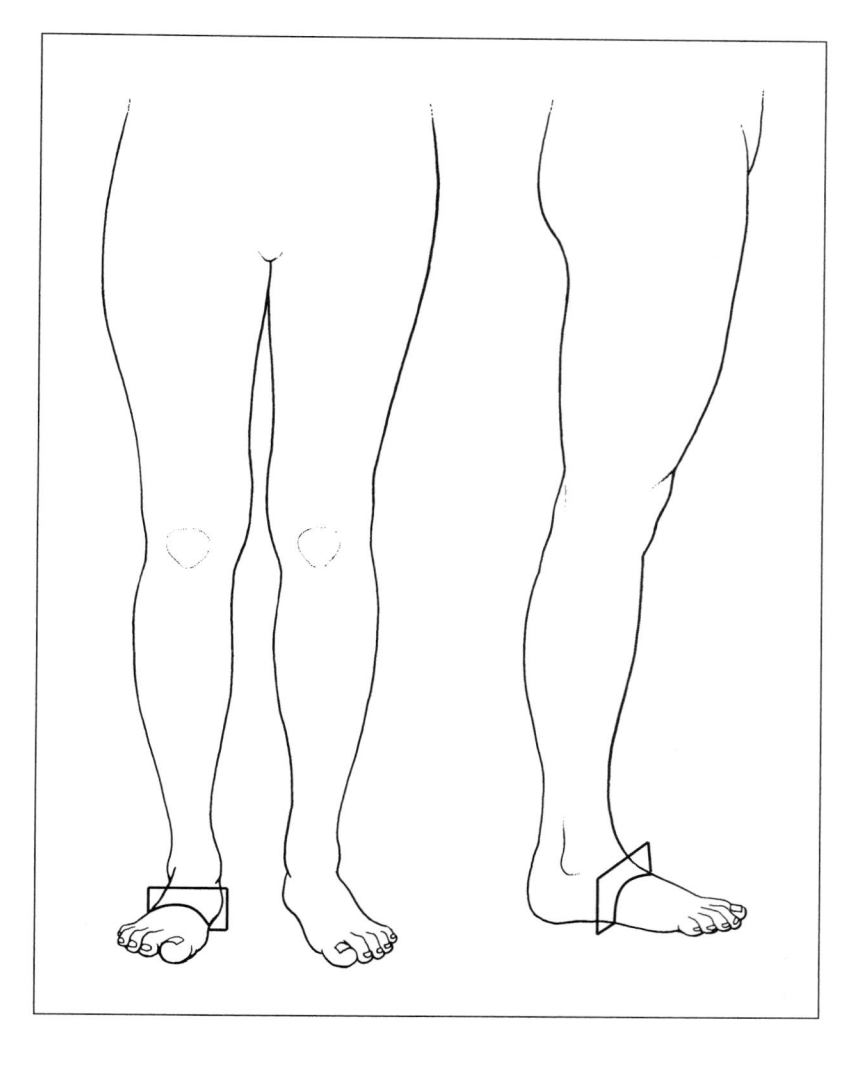

Note

- Compare similarities of the sole of the foot with the palm of the hand (Plate 61).
- The arrangement of the fascia and musculature of the sole into layers is seen ventral to the **three cuneiform bones** (*CN1-CN3*), the **cuboid** (*CB*), and the **base of the 5th metatarsal** (*MT5*).
- The muscle and tendon components of the layers of the sole consist of: (*1*) **superficial fascia** (*SF*), **fat** (*FT*), and the **plantar aponeurosis** (*PA*). In succession, there is (2) a layer of short muscles: **abductor digiti minimi** (*ABM*), **flexor digitorum brevis** (*FDB*), and **abductor hallucis** (*ABH*). (3) The **flexor digitorum longus** (*FDL*) and the **flexor hallucis longus** (*FHL*) and the short muscle, the **quadratus plantae (flexor accessorius)** (*QP*). The adductor hallucis, which also lies in this layer, is farther distal out of this plane of section. (5) **Dorsal** and **plantar interossei** (*IO*) are seen in the deepest layer. The peroneus longus and tibialis posterior are part of this same layer, but have inserted proximal to this plane of section.
- The continuation of the anterior tibial artery, the **dorsalis pedis artery** (*DP*), lies on the dorsum of the foot above the **2nd or middle cuneiform** (*CN2*).
- An **intertarsal joint** (*ITJ*) with its apposing **articular hyaline cartilage** (*CR*) is seen here between the **cuboid bone** (*CB*) and the **3rd or lateral cuneiform** (*CN3*).

Clinical Notes

- Although anatomically somewhat similar, the hand and foot present very clinically distinct problems.
- On imaging, the plantar aspect of the foot has three compartments that are important in isolating and localizing the extent of infection. Medially, there is a compartment containing the muscles of the great toe; laterally, there is a compartment containing the muscles of the small toe. Located centrally are the long flexor tendons and short muscles such as flexor digitorum brevis and quadratus plantae.

References G *5-133 to 5-106;* **N** *500-505;* **RY** *437-439, 467*

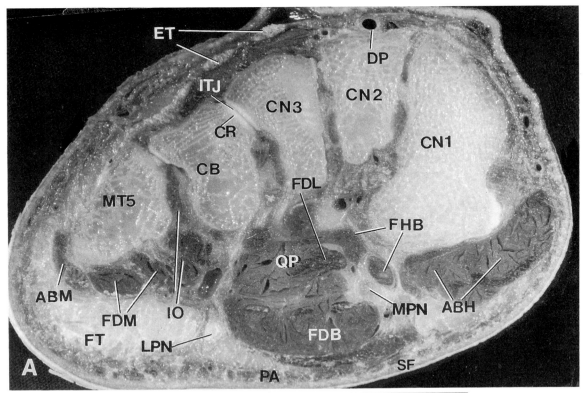

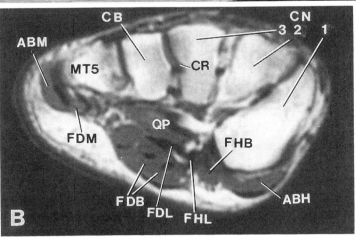

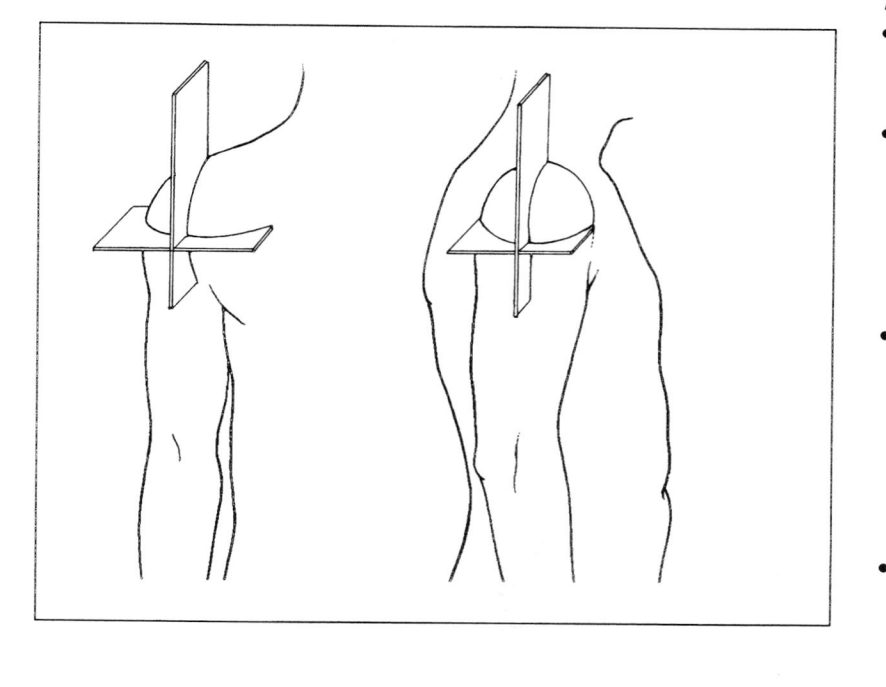

Note

- The transaxial MRI is at least 1.5 cm above the plane of the wet specimen. The coronal wet specimen is in the anatomic position and is more anterior to the coronal oblique plane of the MRI, which is obtained perpendicular to the glenoid fossa.

- The lack of interlocking, supportive bone surfaces is evident in the **shoulder (glenohumeral) joint** (*GHJ*), which presents the relatively small and flat surface of the **glenoid fossa** (*GF*) to the larger surface the **head of the humerus** (*H*), labeled in **A**. The joint surfaces are covered by **hyaline articular cartilage** (*CR*). The **shoulder (glenohumeral) joint** (*GHJ*) is labeled here between its joint surfaces. Note that the wide separation of the joint cavity in **A** and **B** is artifactual. In life, the articular surfaces are closely apposed and are separated only by a thin film of synovial fluid.

- Support involving a set of four "rotator cuff" muscles and their tendons is extremely important. Two of these muscles appear in **A** and **C**. Anteriorly located is the **subscapularis** (*SB*), whose **tendon** (*SBT*) can be seen in **C** to insert anteriorly onto the **lesser tubercle of the humerus** (*LT*). Posteriorly, the **infraspinatus** (*IS*) inserts into the **greater tubercle of the humerus** (*GT*). A third rotator cuff muscle, the **supraspinatus** (*SS*) can be seen in the coronal section in **B**, also inserting into the **greater tubercle** (*GT*). The other rotator cuff muscle is the teres minor, which would be seen in a transaxial section below the plane of the infraspinatus.

- The rotator function of these muscles at the glenohumeral joint is evident from their position. The **subscapularis** (*SB*), inserting anteriorly, rotates the **humerus** (*H*) medially; the **infraspinatus** (*IS*) (and the teres minor), inserting posteriorly, rotates the humerus laterally; **supraspinatus** (*SS*), which runs over the superior side of the joint, initiates abduction of the shoulder joint, allowing a stronger abductor, the **deltoid** (*DL*) to come into play.

Clinical Notes

- The subdeltoid bursa is a potential space that may communicate with the shoulder joint cavity through a rotator cuff tear.

- Complete and partial rotator cuff tears involve the subscapularis tendon in 85% of cases.

- Labral fibrocartilage deepens the shallow bony glenoid fossa and is often torn following dislocation. CT with intra-articular iodinated contrast is still the radiographic standard of reference for glenoid capsule and labral evaluation, although MR imaging is making great strides.

- The subscapularis muscle attaches to the lesser tubercle and is the only rotator cuff muscle that does not attach to the greater tubercle (tuberosity).

References G 6-19 to 6-20, 6-35 to 6-36; **N** 396-398, 400-402; **RY** 356, 400, 349-351, 360-363

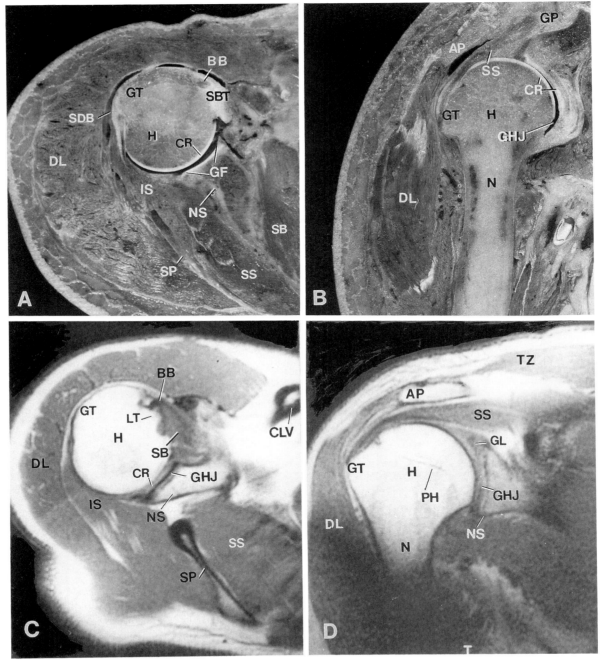

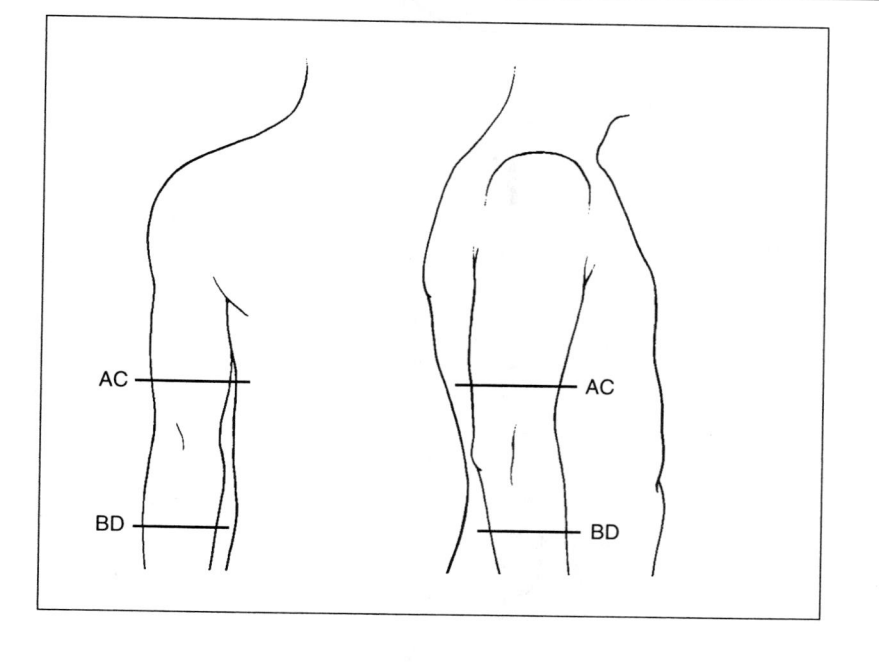

- The compartmentalization of the arm into anterior and posterior compartments, and the forearm into anterior and posterior compartments is indicated in Figures 2B, 19, and 20.

Note

Arm: A and C

- The arm on the MR image **C** is rotated slightly differently from the wet specimen in **A**.
- The arm (**A** and **C**) is divided into anterior and posterior compartments by the **humerus** (*H*) and **medial** and **lateral intermuscular septa** (*LS, MS*). Anterior compartment muscles include the **brachialis** (*BR*), intimately associated with the **humerus** (*H*) and the **biceps brachii** (*BB*). The **musculocutaneous nerve** (*MCN*) is found between these two muscles. The posterior compartment contains the **triceps brachii** (*TCB*), which consists of **lateral** (*LTH*), **medial** (*MH*), and **long heads** (*LOH*). The **radial nerve** (*RN*) lies between the **lateral** and **medial heads** (*LTH, MH*).
- The **ulnar nerve** (*UN*) lies posterior to the **medial intermuscular septum** (*MS*) at this point, and the **median nerve** (*MN*) lies anterior to it on the medial side of the **brachial artery** (*BHA*), close to the **brachial vein** (*BHV*).

Forearm: B and D

- The forearm (**B** and **D**) is irregularly divided into anterior and posterior compartments by the **radius** (*R*) and **ulna** (*U*) and the intervening **interosseous membrane** (*IOM*). In the anterior compartment, superficial, intermediate, and deep sets of muscles are found.
- The **median nerve** (*MN*) occupies a central position deep to the **flexor digitorum superficialis** (*FDS*). The **ulnar nerve** (*UN*), which lies deep to the **flexor carpi ulnaris** (*FCU*), is accompanied by the **ulnar artery** (*UA*) on its medial side. Close to **brachioradialis** (*BD*) is the **superficial radial nerve** (*SRN*), a cutaneous branch of the radial nerve itself, which is accompanied by the **radial artery** (*RA*) on its medial side.
- The posterior compartment is arranged into deep and superficial muscle layers. The superficial muscles number six, three laterally, and three medially and are seen in this plate. The deep muscles are five in number, three of which (all acting on the thumb) are seen here. They are the **abductor pollicis longus** (*ABL*), **extensor pollicis longus** (*EPL*), and the **extensor pollicis brevis** (*EPB*).

Clinical Notes

- The close proximity of the radial nerve to bone makes it vulnerable to injury after fractures of the shaft of the humerus.
- Within the neurovascular bundles, flow phenomena can result in varied appearances of blood vessels. In this example, the higher signal (bright white) may represent slower flow within the vein of the radial neurovascular bundle, associated with dark signal from flow void in different arteries.

References Arm—G 6-39 to 6-44, 6-46 to 6-54; N 396-398, 406-410; RY 364-365, 400; Forearm—G 6-76 to 6-84, 6-122 to 6-123; N 414-423; RY 357, 366-368, 401

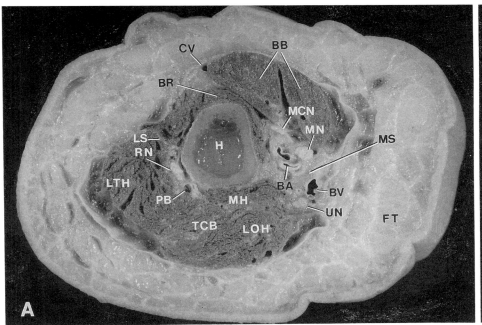

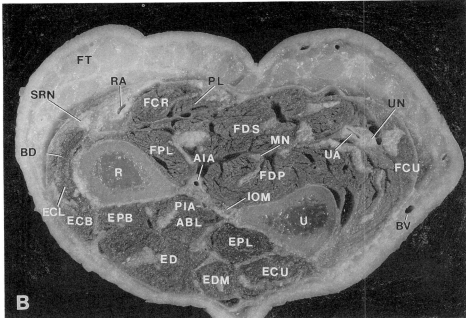

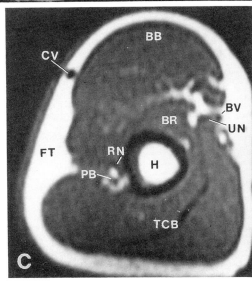

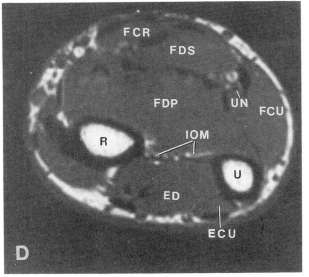

PLATE 59. Elbow joint: transaxial, sagittal, and coronal views: T1 MR images

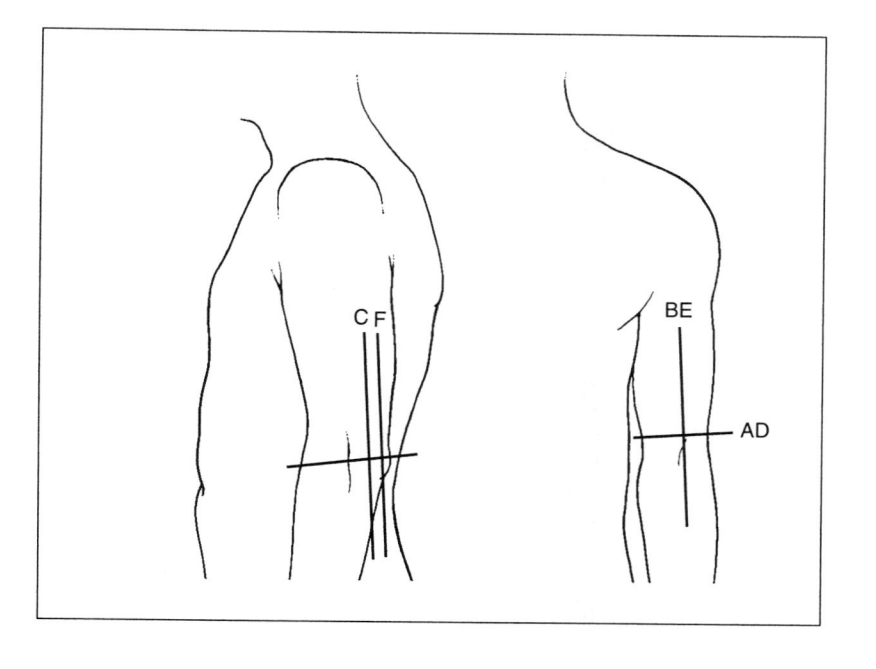

Note

Because of the problem of the semipronated position of the forearm in cadavers, we have opted to present two coronal MR images of the elbow in supination to demonstrate the articulations at the elbow joint. Functionally, these are two in number. One is the elbow joint, made up of the **humeroradial (radiocapitular or radiocapitellar) joint** (*HRJ*) laterally and the **humeroulnar (trochlear ulnar) joint** (*HUJ*) medially. In the latter joint, the coronoid process of the ulna anteriorly and the olecranon process posteriorly have a relationship with the coronoid and olecranon fossae of the humerus in flexion and extension, respectively. The other joint at the elbow is the **proximal radioulnar** (*RUJ*) between the radius and ulna. In addition to movements of flexion, the **humeroradial (radiocapitular) joint** (*HRJ*) also participates with the **proximal radioulnar joint** (*RUJ*) in movements of supination and pronation.

- Many of the nerve, vessel, and muscle relationships can be learned from a study of a transaxial section around the elbow. The **ulnar nerve** (*UN*) lies in a groove posterior to the **medial epicondyle** (*MEP*). The **median nerve** (*MN*), itself posteromedial to the **brachial artery** (*BA*), lies between the **anterior forearm flexors** (*AFM*) and the **brachialis** (*BR*). The **radial nerve** (*RN*) lies between the **brachioradialis** (*BD*) and **brachialis** (*BR*).
- The most important action of **anterior forearm flexors** (*AFM*) is to flex the wrist or the fingers. Similarly, the **posterior forearm extensors** (*EM*) act to extend the wrist or the fingers. A study of figures **A-F** reveals that these muscles are appropriately placed for these roles. Most members of both groups cross the elbow joint after having arisen from common flexor or common extensor tendons attaching respectively to the medial or lateral epicondyles of the humerus.
- The extensors, such as **extensor carpi radialis longus and brevis** (*ECL, ECB*) arise from the common extensor tendon (not seen here), while the **anterior forearm flexors** (*AFM*) arise from the **common flexor tendon** (*CFT*), seen in the MR image in **C**.

Clinical Notes

- Multiplanar imaging is helpful in identifying loose bodies often located in the olecranon recess of the humeroulnar joint.
- Nerve entrapment syndrome involving particularly the ulnar nerve is well evaluated by MR imaging.

References **G** *6-55 to 6-75;* **N** *411-413;* **RY** *357-369, 401*

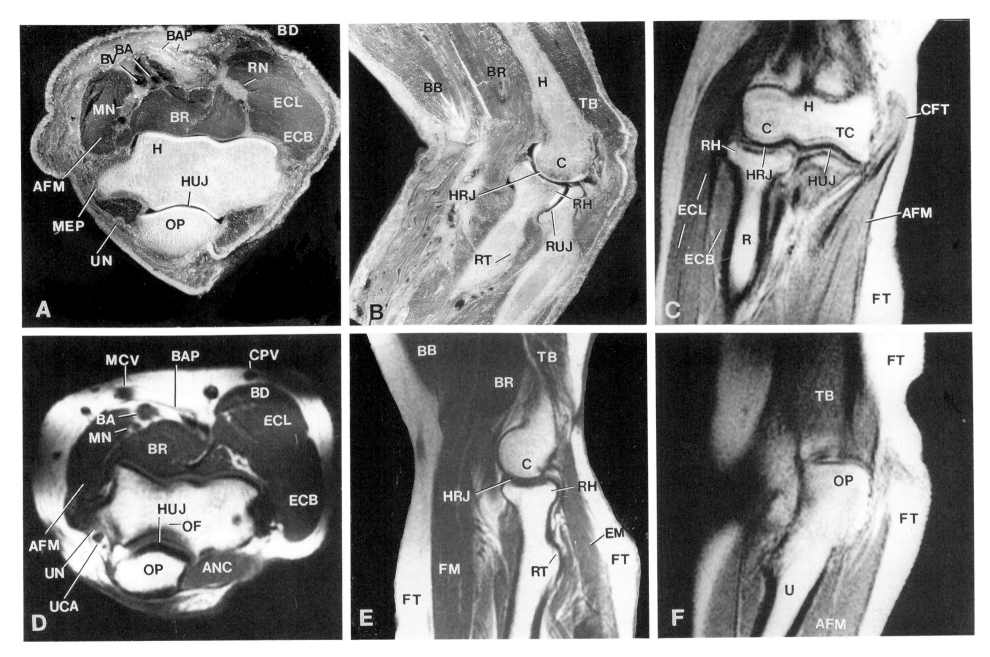

KEY _____

AFM anterior forearm flexors
ANC anconeus
BA brachial artery
BAP bicipital aponeurosis
BB biceps brachii
BD brachioradialis

BR brachialis
BV brachial vein
C capitulum
CFT common flexor tendon
CPV cephalic vein
ECB extensor carpi radialis
  brevis

ECL extensor carpi radialis
  longus
EM extensor muscles of
  forearm
FM anterior forearm flexus
FT subcutaneous fat
H humerus

HRJ humeroradial
  (radiocapitellar) joint
HUJ humeroulnar joint
MCV median cubital vein
MEP medial epicondyle
MN median nerve
OF olecranon fossa

OP olecranon process
R radius
RH head of radius
RN radial nerve
RT radial tuberosity
RUJ proximal radioulnar joint
TB triceps brachii

TC trochlea
U ulna
UCA ulnar collateral artery
  (sup)
UN ulnar nerve

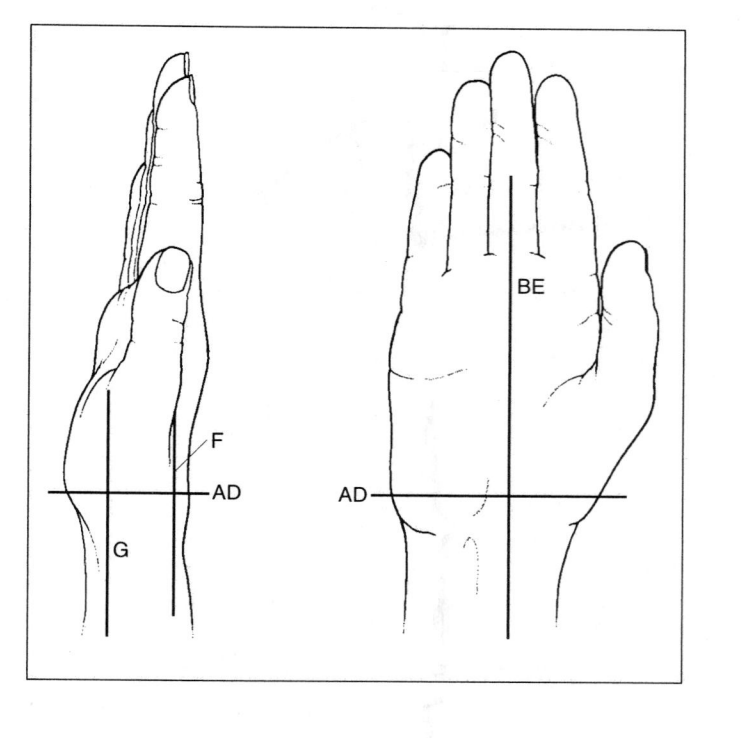

Note

- This plate presents transaxial **A** and **D**, sagittal **B** and **E** and coronal **C**, **F**, and **G** views of the region of the wrist.
- The disposition of carpal bones into a proximal row, **scaphoid** (*SH*), **lunate** (*LU*), **triquetral** (*TQ*), and the more anterior **pisiform** (*PI*), and a distal row **trapezium** (*TM*), **trapezoid** (*TZ*), **capitate** (*CP*), and **hamate** (*HM*) is seen by studying **C**, **F**, and **G**, which present different coronal planes of the wrist.
- In **A** and **D**, the section reveals that the lateral and medial bones are elevated above the central carpal bones forming a carpal tunnel bridged by the **flexor retinaculum** (*FR*). Within this tunnel are the **long flexor tendons of the medial four fingers** (*FT*), **flexor pollicis longus** (*FPL*), and the **median nerve** (*MN*). The position of the tendons relative to proximal and distal rows of carpal bones is seen in **B** and **E** and again in **G**.
- The nature of carpal bones as a link joint between the **radius** (*RA*) and the **metacarpal bones** (*MC1-MC5*) can be understood from **C**, **F**, and **G**. The **midcarpal joint** (*MCJ*) seen here greatly augments movements of the **radiocarpal (wrist) joint** (*RCJ*).
- The passage of vessels into the palm of the hand is revealed in **A** and **D**. In **A**, the **ulnar artery** (*UA*) and **ulnar nerve** (*UN*) pass to the anterolateral side of the **pisiform** (*PI*). Continuing distally, they divide near the **hook of the hamate** (*HK*) (as revealed in **D**) into **deep branches of the ulnar nerve and artery** (*DNA*) and **superficial branches of the ulnar nerve and artery** (*SNA*). The deep branches course into the palm as they pass along the lateral side of the **hook of the hamate** (*HK*). The **radial artery** (*RA*) passes distally alongside the **trapezium** (*TM*) to enter the deep palm.
- The **fibrocartilaginous triangular disk** (*DK*) that separates the **ulna** (*UL*) from the proximal row of carpal bones is seen in **C** and **F**.

Clinical Notes

- Remember that in the anatomical position, the palms face forwards and the thumb is lateral.
- The carpal tunnel syndrome is a well-recognized repetitive stress syndrome. It results from increased pressure of uncertain etiology that secondarily affects the median nerve. It is a common cause of disability in keyboard operators of all kinds. MR can noninvasively define the median nerve and other structures. It is thus used as a problem-solving tool in difficult cases to differentiate other structures passing within the confines of the carpal tunnel.
- A tear of the triangular fibrocartilage or other carpal ligaments is not uncommon. The current standard of reference for diagnosis is the radiographic contrast arthrogram which outlines the joints and follows abnormal movement of injected iodinated contrast.
- Posttraumatic avascular necrosis of the lunate (Keinbock's disease) and of the proximal pole of the scaphoid are recognized by alteration in signal intensity of marrow fat.
- Tendons in T1 MR images have low (dark) signal and often cannot be differentiated from flowing blood, which also has a low (dark) signal secondary to the flow void phenomenon.

References G 6-85 to 6-87, 6-106, 6-126 to 6-136; **N** 426-427; **RY** 358-359, 371

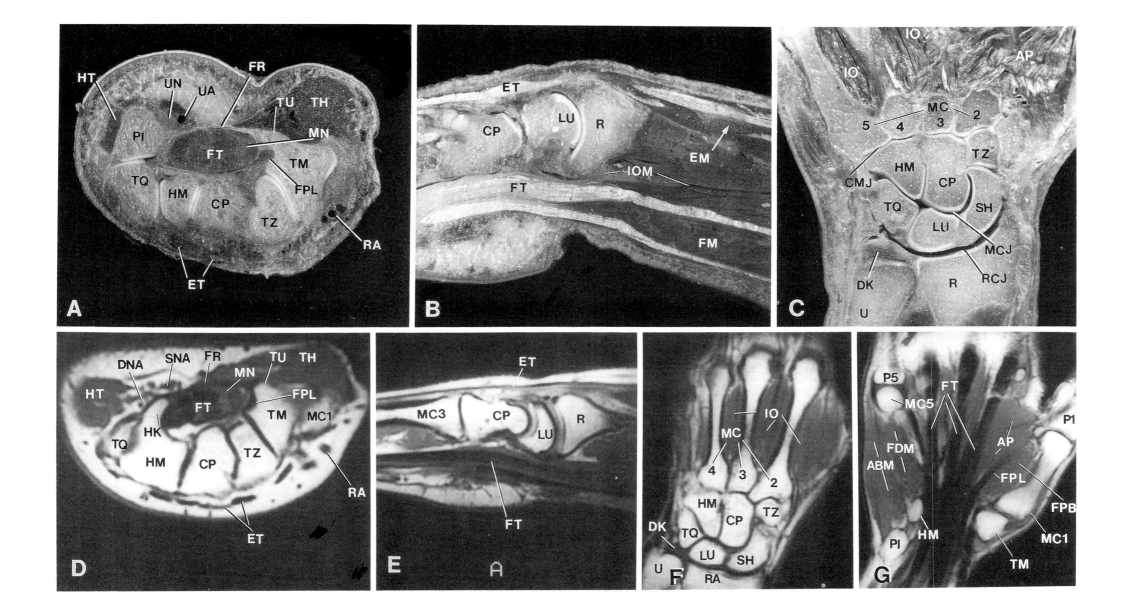

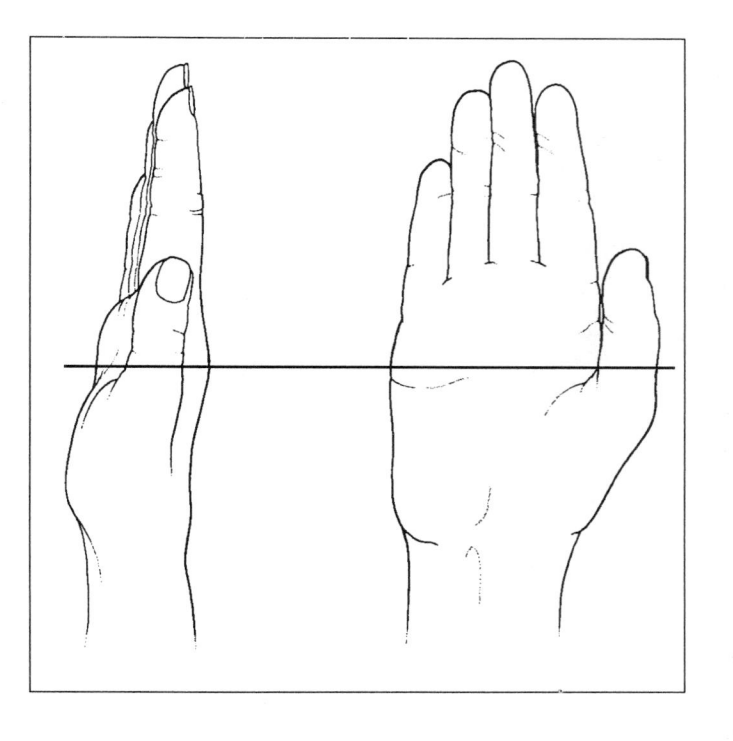

Note

- Compare similarities of the palm of the hand with the sole of the foot (Plate 56).
- The basic arrangement of the palmar fascia and musculature into layers consisting of (*1*) **superficial fascia** (*SF*) and **palmar aponeurosis** (*PA*) in a first layer; (*2*) long tendons of **flexor digitorum superficialis** (*S*) and **flexor digitorum profundus** (*P*), associated with **lumbricals** (*LU*) in a second, slightly deeper layer; (*3*) **dorsal** and **palmar interossei** (*D1-D3, P1-P3*) and the **adductor pollicis** (*AP*) in the deepest central layers of the palm extending as far as the spaces between the **metacarpal bones** (*2-5*).
- The central palm is bordered on its lateral side by a **thenar eminence** (*TE*), which more proximally would be seen to contain three short muscles for the thumb. It is bordered medially by the **hypothenar eminence** (*HTE*), two of whose three short muscles of the little finger appear here (**opponens digiti minimi** [*OPM*] and **abductor digiti minimi** [*ABM*]).
- As previously noted, compact bone gives a darker MRI signal than trabecular bone. This is seen in the **metacarpal bones** (*1-5*), where the outer cortex is dark and the inner marrow cavity with its high content of fat and trabecular bone gives a bright, intermediate signal.
- The long flexor of the thumb, **flexor pollicis longus** (*FPL*), appears adjacent to the **1st metacarpal** (*1*).

Clinical Notes

- The fascial planes of the palm of the hand are not so readily defined by imaging as are the compartments in the leg (see Plate 53).
- The extent of tumor in the muscles planes of the hand and wrist can best be evaluated by MR imaging.
- Developments in local or surface coil technology continue to improve detail in limb imaging.
- Small ganglion cysts, often the source of unexplained soft tissue pain, can also be diagnosed, especially on T2-weighted images.
- Unexplained hand pain of possible osseous origin is usually evaluated initially by radionuclide bone imaging.

References G 6-129, 6-88 to 6-99, 6-129; **N** 431-535; RY 359-370, 401

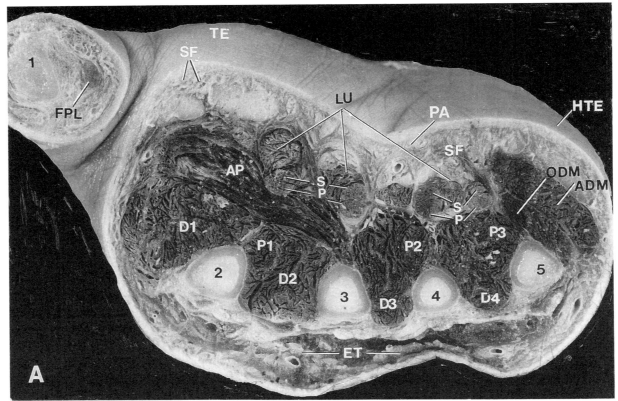

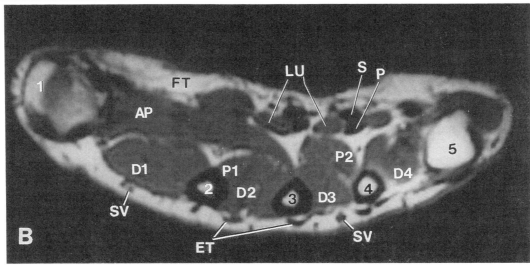

KEY

1–5 metacarpal bones
ADM abductor digiti minimi
AP adductor pollicis

D1–4 dorsal interossei
ET extensor tendons
FPL flexor pollicis longus

FT fat
HTE hypothenar eminence
LU lumbricals

P flexor digitorum profundus
(tendon)
P1–3 palmar interossei

PA palmar aponeurosis
S flexor digitorum superficialis
(tendon)

SF superficial fascia
ODM opponens digiti minimi
SV superficial veins
TE thenar eminence

Index

Please note that, to expedite reference searches, the index lists most terms used in the Primer twice. For example, the sartorius muscle appears as "sartorius muscle" and under the general heading, "muscle, sartorius." The even numbers denote terms identified on plates while odd numbers denote terms used in the plate descriptions.

126

130